Master the Art of Running

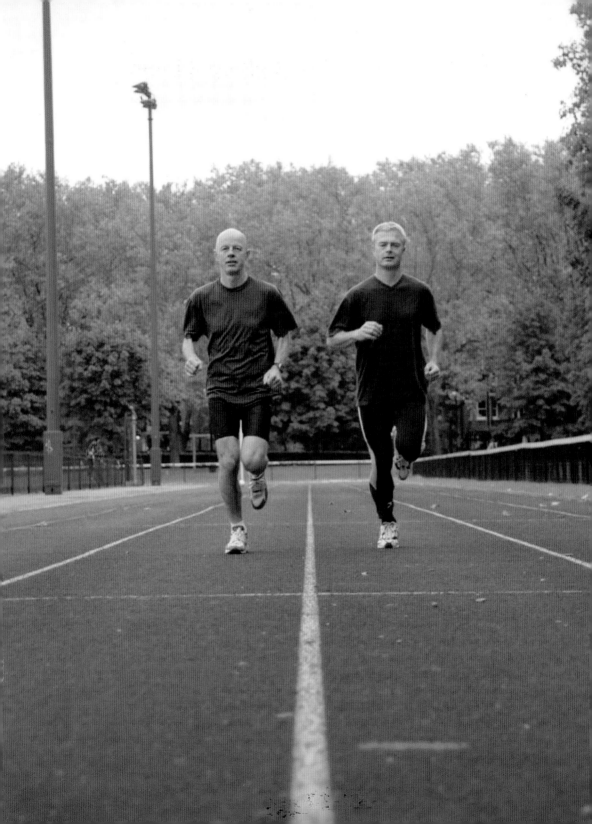

Malcolm Balk and Andrew Shields

Master the Art of Running

Raise Your Performance with the Alexander Technique

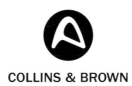

COLLINS & BROWN

First published in the United Kingdom in 2006
This edition first published in 2009 by
Collins & Brown
10 Southcombe Street
London, W14 0RA

An imprint of Anova Books Company Ltd

ISBN 978-1-84340-543-6

A CIP catalogue for this book is available from the British
Library.

10 9 8 7 6 5 4 3 2 1

Reproduction by Anorax Imaging Ltd
Printed and bound by 1010 Printing International Limited,
China

Keep updated. Email sales@anovabooks.com for FREE
email alerts on forthcoming titles.

www.anovabooks.com

To the spirit and legacy of Terry Fox

To all the runners I have trained with, competed against
and worked with, thanks for helping me become a better
runner, coach and person.

To my fellow Alexander teachers for their interest and
encouragement, inparticular: Jean Clark, Steven Cooper,
Liz Dodgson, Jonathan Drake, Brita Forsstrom, Arie Jan
Hoorweg, Carolyn Nichols, Merran Poplar, Roy Palmer,
Maggie Rakusen, Steven Shaw, Robin Simmons, Ken
and Angela Thompson, Paul Versteeg and Tessa
Marwick, and John Woodward. Particular thanks to
Dr Nicholas Romanov, originator of the Pose Method of
running, for his ability to think outside the box and inspire
a new generation of runners. To Marilyn Arsenault,
thanks for working with me on the Pose Method. To
Dave and Tina for a base on the Grove.

A very special thanks to my wife Pamela and 2020
Olympic 800 m champion, my son Milo. **Malcolm Balk**

To Mark Harrod, Roger Mallett and Brigitte Wrenn of
Central YMCA for support and forbearance, particularly
when important keys end up on the wrong side of the
Atlantic. To Julia Armstrong and fellow coaches with the
London Active Partnership and Ilford Athletic Club,
thanks for your encouragement and stimulating
discussions.

Particular thanks to my endlessly patient wife Elaine and
children Helen, Isabel and Matthew. **Andrew Shields**

Both authors would like to thank those runners who
contributed case studies to this book. Also Brad
Thompson of Ashgrove Publishing for his commitment to
our original vision of 'The Art of Running', and Katie
Cowan and Victoria Alers-Hankey at Anova Books for
their ongoing creative and technical support.

CONTENTS

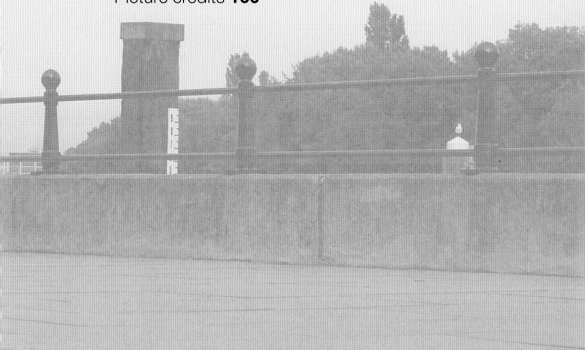

INTRODUCTION

'Running is the greatest metaphor for life, because you get out of it what you put into it.' Oprah Winfrey

Why do we run? First and foremost, we run because it gives us pleasure. It makes us feel good – about ourselves, and about the world in general. We run to enjoy the feeling of movement, to overcome inertia, to begin to flow. We run to do battle with our demons, real and imagined. We run to improve our fitness and well-being. We run to transcend the elements, to renew ourselves, to connect with the beauty and energy and vibrancy of life. Some of us run to compete, and maybe to win.

Staying present

Every run should be different, and the way we react to each run can be a matter of choice or creation. For example, when I ran today, I noticed that my right hamstring felt tight. As I ran, I kept monitoring my leg and also noticed how it was affecting my overall form. It caused me to tighten my back and run more heavily than I wished. So I decided to stop and give my body some direction. I pointed myself upwards, encouraged my knees and ankles to release, and started again. Soon my stride was smoother and I was breathing more freely. A distance of 100 m (328 ft) further on, I stopped again to repeat the process. Picking up the pace, I noticed that my hamstring was starting to release, but still gave me an occasional twinge. I continued, but later, as I was doing some accelerations, I noticed that my hamstring had let go and was now part of my overall sense of falling upwards and forwards. I pressed on with the day's workout, taking care not to let its demands overwhelm my kinaesthetic ear and my decision to flow rather than force my way through each repetition.

I have completed a version of that workout many times, but today it was an experience that demanded my creative intelligence just to do it. It was an illustration of running as an act of creativity: staying present,

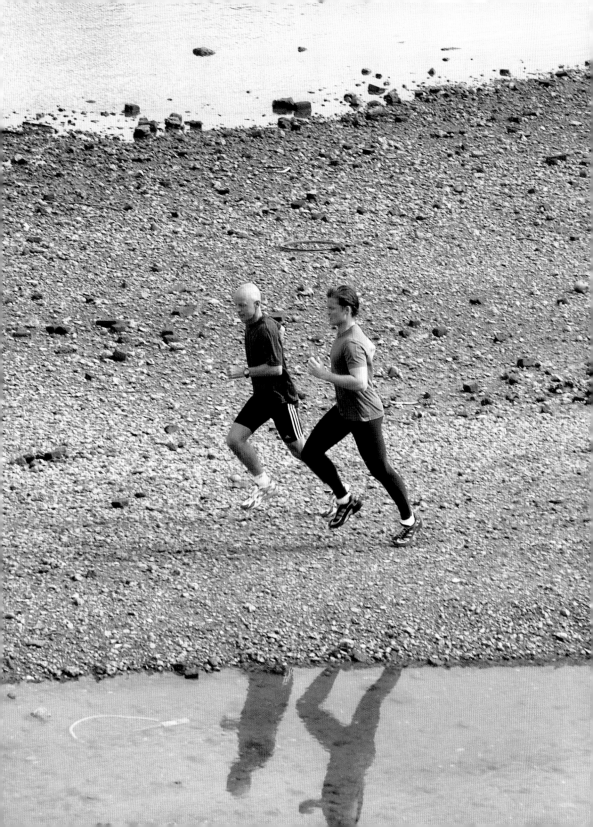

responding thoughtfully to the situation, taking calculated risks, and finding a different way to achieve your goal.

For some people, however, running can become tedious – just another item to be ticked off on the list of the day's tasks. And when any activity becomes routine, no matter what it is, boredom and blindness set in and we wish we were somewhere else doing something more exciting.

One sign that an activity is becoming routine is a tendency to distance yourself from what you are doing. 'Distance' doesn't mean the healthy detachment that allows you to see what is going on with greater clarity, less interference and more control. Rather it's the semi-comatose, trance-like state we can easily slide into, especially when we are doing something we've done a thousand times before. Who doesn't remember the thrill of getting behind the wheel of a car for the first time, putting it into gear and steering uncertainly round an empty car park. Is driving anything like that today?

When running becomes just a means to an end – whether that's fitness, fame or fat reduction – it loses the features that elevate it from being just another mundane activity. When we cut our minds off from what we are doing and simply mechanically repeat a movement over and over again, without interest or curiosity, without thought and without intention, we reduce both the experience and ourselves in the process. We are no longer immersed in the moment. Instead, we simply want to 'get it done'. As Oprah says in the quotation at the start of this chapter, running is there for us to do with as we please. We can approach it with enthusiasm and zest, eager to see each run as an opportunity for learning and self-discovery. Or we can approach it half-heartedly, reluctant to push ourselves physically and emotionally, content to stay within the confines of previous experience. It's the latter group, uncertain of what they are doing and why, who become bored and uninspired and tend to give up.

The art of running

Is running boring? It can be – if you let it. It is far better to approach running as an art, with skills to be learned and practised. The art of running is to be found in the process, and it needs to be recreated every time you run. It doesn't matter what you did yesterday, or even what you did two minutes ago – it's always the next step that counts. The quality of the experience is what matters most.

The Alexander Technique

When running is approached as an art, rather than as a technique, a science or a means to fitness, it takes on a whole new dimension. First of all, the runner's motivation changes. The emphasis is less on targets such as winning a race or breaking a preordained time, and more on the process of exploration and enhanced awareness that running offers. That is the theme of this book, which is underpinned by the principles of the Alexander Technique, developed by Frederick Alexander. The Technique is a method for teaching us how to develop conscious control over our reactions, which can be the source of unproductive and involuntary patterns of movement and behaviour. These automatic reactions are habits that we fall into without thinking – the most fundamental being a tendency to pull the head back and down and thus distort the balanced relationship between the head, neck and back. The Technique teaches us to reassert effective command over the way we think and act, helping to unlearn the habits of a lifetime. Through this psychophysical reintegration, we can begin to get back in touch with our selves. For runners, the benefits are obvious.

Alexander also believed that when we become overly preoccupied with results, we lose touch with the process. He called this 'end-gaining'. It's an attitude so widespread in our society that it is almost 'normal' (although certainly not natural). Getting back in touch with the process puts us in the moment, and each moment is a little different from the one before it.

Assuming that we know how to run, for example, is one way of stopping what should be an ongoing process of learning and discovery. Perhaps you have been running for fifteen to twenty years and you are absolutely certain that you know what you're doing. Yet this kind of thinking leaves you bankrupt, as far as learning goes. All runners, even the very best,

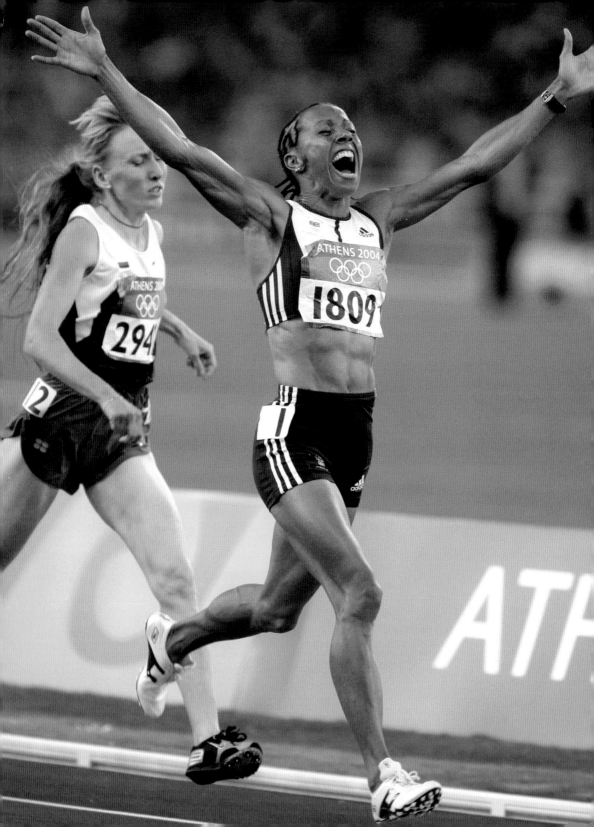

have something that could be improved or changed. A willingness to let go, then find anew, is central to the art of running.

Just as musicians, dancers, actors, artists and gymnasts practise, so do athletes. Kelly Holmes won the 2004 Olympic 800 m and 1500 m finals in 1 min 56 secs and 3 mins 57 secs respectively, but it took her fifteen years of practice to do so: time spent partly in the company of fellow runners but mostly by herself, repeating drills and training routines over and over again while striving to keep each workout fresh and meaningful. What can we lesser mortals bring to our practice that will elevate it from the level of mindless repetition?

Mastering the basics is important for enjoying the process. Learning to run takes time, energy and consistency: you have to do it regularly to become good at it. And until you've achieved a certain level of competence, it can be difficult to enjoy. Some runners are unwilling to believe that there is something new to be learned every time they lace up their shoes, but the fact is, it's true. Being curious about what we are doing is another key ingredient – otherwise everything gets old, stale and lifeless. If world and Olympic champions admit that they could have run faster if they'd had a better start, or had been more relaxed or more focused, then the rest of us can certainly find something to discover, change or improve.

◀ **KELLY HOLMES**
*The great British middle-distance athlete won the 2004
Olympic 800 m and 1,500 m titles in 1 min 56 secs and 3 min
57 secs respectively, but it took her 15 years of practice to
do so – a time spent striving to keep each workout fresh
and meaningful.*

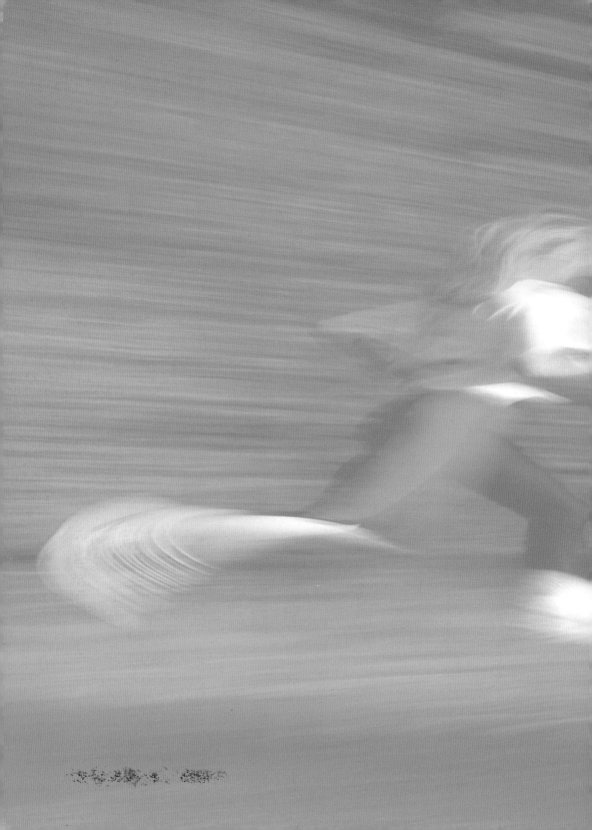

1

THE ART OF RUNNING

'We run because we enjoy it and cannot help ourselves. The more restricted our society and work become, it will be necessary to find some outlet for this craving for freedom. No one can say you must not run faster than this, or jump higher than that. The human spirit is indomitable.'

Sir Roger Bannister

Muhammad Ali's claim to 'float like a butterfly, sting like a bee' is more than a great quotation. It encapsulates the fact that the world's most famous boxer could not have unleashed so many telling punches without having superb balance, poise, grace, efficiency and kinaesthetic awareness. Ali was a magnificent example of an athlete possessed of something which, in the Alexander Technique, is known as 'good use'.

We can all appreciate such perfect form, whether it's displayed by a boxer, footballer, swimmer, gymnast, athlete or dancer. Think of Haile Gebrselassie or any number of other African runners, Torville and Dean, Fred Astaire, Carl Lewis, Ronaldo, Ian 'Thorpedo' Thorpe, Margot Fonteyn or Mikhail Baryshnikov: these sportspeople and performers make the impossible look easy.

It is common to hear sports and exercise professionals describe athletes as having 'good mechanics'. By this they usually mean someone who demonstrates a high level of skill, has excellent technique and who moves smoothly and efficiently. This is a subject which can get seriously complicated: read just a little about how biomechanists describe technique and you're into kinematics and kinetics, appropriate forces being applied in the right direction, muscles firing in the correct combinations and sequences, and so on.

We are right to pay such close attention to form, so let's keep it simple. After all, it's fair to assume that most of us don't just want to run for a few weeks, but to continue running in a sustainable way once the original euphoria has worn off. Furthermore, we know that exercising in an uncoordinated and inefficient manner increases the risk of injury.

At the heart of the Alexander Technique is a belief that 'use' affects functioning. In other words, it's vital to consider how we do things, not just what we do. For some people, merely lacing up their trainers is a major accomplishment, while actually getting out on the street and running for twenty minutes may be cause for major celebration. However, for those who run regularly but find their fitness levels reaching a plateau and notice an increase in persistent niggles, the issue is more serious. This is why it's important to pay attention to use.

Talent, technique and use

'Talent' is what we're born with. It's our potential. 'Technique' is the know-how needed to perform a movement or activity. 'Use' is the way we do things, with specific awareness of the relationship between our head, neck and back. The three concepts are not synonymous.

Some people can fall out of bed with a stinking hangover and still run 10 km (6 miles) or do the splits as if it's no big deal. Many sportspeople, including athletes, don't have particularly good use yet have developed high levels of skill in their particular activity. For example, footballers may hunch their backs and tighten their shoulders, but despite 'misusing' themselves in these ways, they can still control a ball with great skill and precision. In contrast, a person can have 'good use' but lack the technique or skill needed to throw a javelin, leap over hurdles or execute a triple jump.

Is there a link between good use and good form? Sometimes, but not always. Take the example of alignment. We are often urged to think about showing 'proper alignment' when we exercise. This usually means stacking things up on top of each other so we are in better balance. If a coach encourages you to keep your back straight, most people assume that they can do it, and that their idea of 'straight' is correct. This isn't always so: ask a friend to stand straight (that is, vertically) and nine times out of ten you'll find that he tends to lean backwards. He'll also be prepared to swear that when he stands against a wall, he is leaning forwards. So how does a coach correct this situation? Often with well-intentioned yet potentially harmful advice such as 'Pull in your belly button', 'Tighten your buttocks', 'Pull your shoulders back' or 'Pull in your chin'. It's the classic 'outside-in' approach loved by army drill sergeant-majors the world over and shows that what is conventionally thought of as 'proper alignment' can only be achieved at considerable expense.

Use implies freedom, and freedom is a condition, not a position. On the track, some people look good, but their bodies betray great rigidity; their joints are stiff, so whatever they try and do requires more effort than the results warrant. This is an example of good alignment with poor use.

As a competitive athlete, I wished for more natural talent because there were some aims that, no matter how much I trained and sharpened my fitness level, I was never able to achieve. For example, I trained for and competed in the 800 m for ten years with the hope of breaking a time of two minutes, a goal I never accomplished. Yet I have coached runners who broke this time in their first year, often with poor technique and bad use.

So where does this leave us? Talent is something that we all have to some degree. We don't have any say in the amount of talent that we're blessed with, but bad use will undoubtedly limit our ability to develop it fully. However, technical skill can be learned and good use can be worked on and improved. They are both within our sphere of influence. I didn't have the God-given talent to break two minutes in the 800 m, but I did manage to run 2:04. This was a faster time than I would have been able to achieve if I hadn't trained (developed my potential) or, equally importantly, if I hadn't applied the principles of the Alexander Technique to the process.

If you don't have the genetic make-up to be a world-class athlete, swimmer, dancer or gymnast, no amount of good use will make you one. It's the same when it comes to training: some people are born to sprint with ease, others to complete a marathon and barely break sweat. For we lesser mortals, the Alexander Technique and its principle of good use will enhance any activity to which it is applied. It makes it easier to assimilate new skills and helps us develop our potential. And it makes the whole business of learning a lot less painful and much more fun.

Models of fitness

Inactivity is unhealthy, but activity can be unhealthy too. When I was running marathons in the late 1970s, I affected a degree of bravado not uncommon among those who punish themselves in the quest for peak performance. The fact that I was injured on a regular basis, caught more than my share of colds and looked like I'd been suffering from chronic dysentery was neither here nor there. I was a 'marathoner' – case closed. I viewed people who refused to match my level of commitment as slightly pathetic. Should they deign to do a little running as a means of staying fit (in a sensible, planned and realistic 'healthy' sense), I quickly dismissed them as mere joggers. Without question, I confused being fit – meaning 'fit to compete' – with being healthy.

This is an unintelligent attitude, which ignores the purpose and process of exercise and is obsessed with end results, denying the possibility of finding an approach that satisfies one's whole self in favour of the quick fix. After all, if we feel that something is wrong in our lives, isn't it foolish to try and redress the balance with something that's equally wrong? It helps to explain why new gym memberships peak in January as hordes of overindulgers throw themselves into the fitness regime they pledged in a drunken stupor on New Year's Eve – with most 'converts' back in their armchairs three months later.

Let's be honest: one of the main reasons we run and work out is to look good. This is especially true if, as we get older, our internal sense of youthful vitality still corresponds to some degree with the exterior bodywork!

The 'SMART' approach to running

In October 2002, *The Times* ran a feature entitled 'A Day in the Life of an Exercise Bike', in which the twenty-five people who used a particular machine in a fitness club were interviewed about their motivations and goals. All were reasonably regular attendees and their attitude to working out was generally favourable: 'I love it', 'If I don't come I get really depressed', 'Love it once I'm here', 'I tell myself off for not coming more often'. However, their responses when asked about 'cycling thoughts' were also of a type: 'I usually switch off', 'My mind goes totally blank', 'I think what the hell are we all doing?', 'What's next on MTV?', 'Without TV, magazines and books I'd be bored', 'Anything but the pain', 'I usually blank out'. In fact, not one of them mentioned paying attention to the activity they were performing – which is revealed by the hunched shoulders and tight necks in the accompanying photographs. Even though all claimed to enjoy using the gym and recognized the physical benefits, their minds were elsewhere – or nowhere at all.

The interviewer would probably have gained similar responses from twenty-five users of a treadmill. Or, by standing on a street corner, twenty-five joggers – many, no doubt, plugged into an iPod and using music as a distraction from the activity they were engaged in. All these people are keen enough to run or work out, but clearly lack the focus needed to exercise with purpose. They would benefit from the 'SMART' approach, to prevent the wrong things happening right from the start – it is the key to running and working out successfully, effectively and enjoyably.

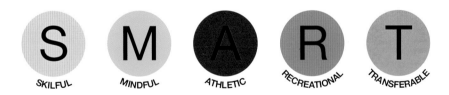

S = Skilful

The idea that one can perform any activity with skill, grace and courage is barely considered by most people. While your fitness level will obviously play a role in how you 'perform', it is not the only – or even the primary – reason for the dismal form displayed by many runners. John Jerome describes this poignantly:

One reason we have pets is for the enjoyment of being surrounded by such great, natural athletes. (Compared to an ordinary house cat, Mikhail Baryshnikov is a stumblebum.) On a recent morning, though, I noticed that the older dog, Molly, was a little tentative, not moving very well. She did a surprisingly bad job of leaping over a small brook – and then I, following, did a bad job of it too. It made me realize that I was moving all hunched up, unsure, tense. I wasn't warmed up yet but that was no excuse. What I was really seeing was that Molly was moving like an old dog and that I was moving like an old man. Stop it, I told myself. Stop running like a doddering old gaffer. I managed to do it for 50 yards or so, but then my shoulders were up around my ears again. I have a terrible time remembering to stay loose, but then I'm not much of an athlete.

John Jerome, *The Elements of Effort*

M = Mindful

'I'm so poor I can't even pay attention.' (That's a joke, by the way.) For example, when you're in the gym doing some cross-training and are lifting a weight, do you focus solely on the part of the body that's doing the work? Or are you aware of the way that lifting the weight is affecting the rest of you? Are you stiffening your neck, clenching your teeth, distorting your back and holding your breath? Are you still aware of what's going on around you, or have you blinded yourself to your environment? Do you know what the proper technique is for what you're doing and do you employ it? Are you interested in what you're doing or are you off in the clouds somewhere? Back to running: do you move smoothly or do you tend to jerk, plod and pound – anything to complete the damn run! – particularly when you start to get tired?

A = Athletic

Here are two stereotypes you might find on the treadmill next to you. There's the man who muscles his way through every routine, tackling tough hill climbs with gritted teeth and pounding along at an excessive speed (you can hear his feet hammering down on the surface from outside the room), regardless of how this is affecting his overall use and unwilling to take advice from an instructor. And there's the woman who runs so slowly and timidly that it's unlikely the process is providing any benefit whatsoever.

One doesn't have to be born with the genetic make-up of an athlete to start acting like one. On the other hand, even someone with physical talents can start to look feeble with poor use, their athletic ability totally hidden when slouched in a chair or standing casually with hips thrust forwards, lower back arched and neck tight. But when the head leads and the body follows in a careful and coordinated manner, simple movements such as bending to pick something up, getting out of a chair, climbing stairs or lifting a child can take on the grace, skill, power and coordination of more 'athletic' activities.

R = Recreational

'Recreation' is defined in the dictionary as 'refreshment of one's mind or body after labour through diverting activity: play!' For many people, running has become just another job, something else to tick off on the endless list of things to do. We need to remember that all-important sense of fun, and keep a sense of perspective about our training programmes.

T = Transferable

If we view running and working out as more than just a means of enhancing the aesthetic (such as developing 'six-pack' abs) and look at its wider applications, then we must include the notion that training should be transferable to our daily existence – what is now termed 'functional fitness'. But here's the rub: many of the movements and routines performed in the gym are not normally found in nature. They are merely creations of the gym environment. For example, in everyday life, when do you ever move your arms in the motion prescribed by the pec-deck?

Finally, if we assume that good use is the gold standard towards which any runner should aspire, good use according to the principle of specificity should be practised in every workout. Otherwise we run the risk of perfecting – that is, further ingraining – our bad habits rather than cultivating good ones.

You and your body

Whatever level athletes compete at, they talk of being 'in the zone' – when body and mind are in such perfect connection that a great performance flows effortlessly. Jockeys, too, describe moments when it seems as though they and their mount are as one, and the rider's wishes are immediately sensed and responded to by the animal. Driving, tennis, archery, skiing and golf are among the other activities where people have experienced this inspiring effect.

Sometimes, however, a belief in one's own unity of body and mind can be given a severe jolt. I will never forget the time I took a group of boys from a youth club on a pony trekking expedition. I was given what I took to be an intelligent animal called Ernst. But no matter what I did, Ernst ignored me and carried on walking after the lead pony. Yelling, kicking and pleading did nothing to improve matters. This joyless arrangement culminated in Ernst taking me under a tree branch which he cleared easily but which caused me, much to the delight of the boys, to be knocked to the ground as it hit me in the chest. I was very glad to return to base and bid Ernst farewell (and wish him an untimely trip to the animal food processing plant). To rub salt into the wound of my bruised ego and bottom, many of the boys (to whom I was supposed to provide some sort of example) seemed to have a wonderful rapport with their mounts and could coax them into changing direction or gait with little or no effort.

There's a lesson here, since this incident resembles the relationship some of us have with running. Is there a way to improve our relationship with, and ultimately the functioning of, our selves? Are willpower and a regular training regime enough to bring about change – or is something else required?

What is fitness?

In a purely physical sense, fitness is the ability of the heart, lungs, circulatory system and muscles to function at optimum efficiency. However, this is a very limited definition. As we have seen, we must always consider the transferability of our physical activity to daily life. This means asking the question: fit for what?

If you are training for a marathon or an Ironman triathlon, your answer will be very different to that of someone who wants to start gentle jogging to lose weight, or someone who is recovering from a long spell in hospital after surgery. Fitness is the ability to carry out a given task effectively and safely. For elite athletes, that means being ready to compete at the highest level; for the majority of us, it means being fit to live our lives with vigour. As Rodney Cullum and Lesley Mowbray put it in *The YMCA Guide to Exercise to Music*: 'Total fitness includes physical, nutritional, medical, mental, emotional and social fitness. It can be described as the ability to meet the needs of the environment, plus a little in reserve for emergencies.'

However, the art of running is to strive for a far higher ideal of fitness than any of its parts. 'It is a state of being rather than doing,' add Cullum and Mowbray, 'and available to all regardless of skill level, movement quality, body type, sex or any other heredity or environmental influence.' The aim is to live with an enriched quality of life rather than to merely exist. 'If total fitness is your aim, you will have to develop an independence of attitude that makes you self-reliant; you will exercise because you value fitness, not because you are told to exercise.' This independence of thought and a willingness to 'think in activity' are central to the art of running.

Models of running

The Alexander Technique, as we will discover in more detail in Chapter 2, does not tell us how to run, how to play the cello or how to perform any other skilled activity. It simply informs the process. To learn how to run, there are existing models to which we can refer. These show how different coaches have approached the subject, producing a variety of techniques which at times contradict each other. Here are some examples:

The 'default' or 'natural' approach

Supporters of this approach believe that everyone has a unique gait or stride pattern, developed from the time we begin to walk. The 'default' approach proposes that changing (and therefore improving) this gait is next to impossible. This means that when a person wants to improve, or encounters an injury, change has to be made 'from the outside in'. In other words, physiotherapy, orthotics, supportive shoes and trying harder!

For average runners who are either not aware of or not interested in changing/improving their manner of running, i.e. their form, this approach is probably as good as it gets. If you are born with good use and have strong connective tissue, along with a liberal sprinkling of natural talent, it's an approach that can be extremely effective!

A frequent discussion point among runners is why Kenyans run so well. First of all, it needs to be stated that not all Kenyans run well. Those who do tend to come

THE FIVE COMPONENTS OF FITNESS

- **Cardiovascular fitness**, otherwise known as stamina, endurance or aerobic fitness. This is the efficiency of the heart, lungs and circulatory system: improvements that produce a 'training effect'.

- **Muscular strength**, or the ability of a muscle to exert sufficient force to overcome a resistance. By increasing the resistance, the muscle is trained to work more efficiently.

- **Muscular endurance** or the ability of muscles to overcome the resistance for a prolonged period of time.

- **Flexibility**, to lengthen the muscles and increase the range of movement of the joints.

- **Motor fitness**, which includes such factors as agility, balance, reaction time, coordination, power and speed.

from specific regions of the country and have a lifestyle in which running plays a major role; the environmental conditions are also conducive to running. Indeed, it has been said that the difference between an 18-year-old Kenyan runner and his Canadian counterpart is 30,000 km (18,642 miles)! If that is what this school means by 'natural', there is no argument from us!

Unfortunately, the average Western runner is not only way behind the starting line but 'enjoys' a lifestyle that is largely sedentary and not conducive to good natural running. Consider the Zen saying, 'Wherever you go, there you are!'. If you sit, stand and move with bad use, there's a pretty strong chance you will bring those same damaging qualities to your running. But here's where we part company with the determinist school of running. These conditions are not immutable, not fixed for life. They can be changed – something Alexander Technique practitioners experience every day.

Implication for runners: *improve your use and you will improve your running, whichever approach you subscribe to.*

The heel-toe approach

This is probably the most widely practised and recommended technique for runners at all levels, right up to elite competitors. Its guiding principle is this: land on the heel, roll through the foot and push off with the toes. There is an interesting and not unsurprising similarity between the heel-toe approach and the 'default' model. Just as, for most people, the act of sitting drops to the lowest common denominator and becomes the act of slumping, running seems to follow suit and becomes more of a shuffle than a stride.

Recommended on the grounds of both safety and efficiency, the heel-toe method, upon closer examination, proves to be neither. In spite of endless innovations and improvements in shoe technology, the number and frequency of running injuries have remained constant over the last thirty years. Since most people run heel-toe, there is at least correlative evidence that this may not be the safest way to run. In terms of efficiency, here's what Michael Yessis has to say:

If you are a heel hitter and land with the sole of your foot angled upward, you will experience braking forces on each touchdown. This means that each time your heel hits the ground it breaks your forward momentum and can generate extremely high forces – from two- to ten-times body weight depending on the angle of the foot and contact, and the speed of running. In general, the greater the angle of the foot when the heel hits the ground and the greater the speed of running, the greater the forces generated.

Michael Yessis, *Explosive Running*

Because the heel strike is erroneously considered 'natural', footwear companies make running shoes with a well-cushioned heel to absorb the landing forces. From a biomechanical standpoint, this cushioning (and the heel lift) is not only very inefficient but works against the natural muscle and tendon functions. In fact, some recent studies on running shoes indicate that they may be a major culprit in running injuries. Holy conspiracy theory, Batman! Some of these issues are explored later in this book.

Implication for runners: *just because they say it's 'tried and true' doesn't mean it is!*

The competitive approach

Not every runner is interested in competing on the track, road or in cross-country, but for those who are, the competitive approach has a lot of appeal. It is best described in the book *Winning Running* by Peter Coe, father of double Olympic gold medallist Sebastian Coe. It is characterized by a strong push, including the toe-off, an explosive knee drive and powerful arm action.

Implication for runners: *not for everyone, especially those over forty.*

Pose and Chi running approaches

Nicholas Romanov is a Russian coach who has pioneered what is known as the Pose Method of running. An innovative thinker whose work has received much interest, particularly among triathletes, Romanov believes that it would be better if we learned to use gravity as the primary source of power in running. By learning how to collaborate skilfully with gravity, running becomes more efficient with less reliance on muscular effort to propel us towards our destination.

Pose Method differs from the other models in that the emphasis is on falling and getting the support off the ground rather than pushing off with the toes and driving forwards with the knee. Pose Method teaches human movement by determining its key pose, or position, and focusing primarily on this. In running, this is a whole-body pose where the shoulders, hips and ankles are vertically aligned with the support leg, while balancing on the forefoot. This creates an S-shape in the leg. The support foot is pulled from the ground as the runner falls forwards, while the other foot drops down freely

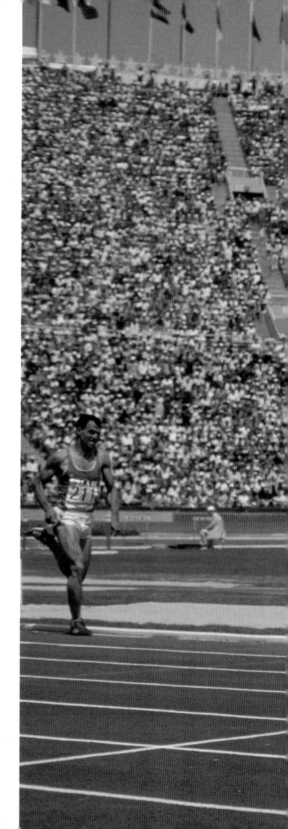

ED MOSES ▶

400 m hurdles legend Ed Moses at full extension – a magnificent example of his ability to maintain direction longer than his competitors. Note the strong toe-off, explosive knee drive and powerful arm action.

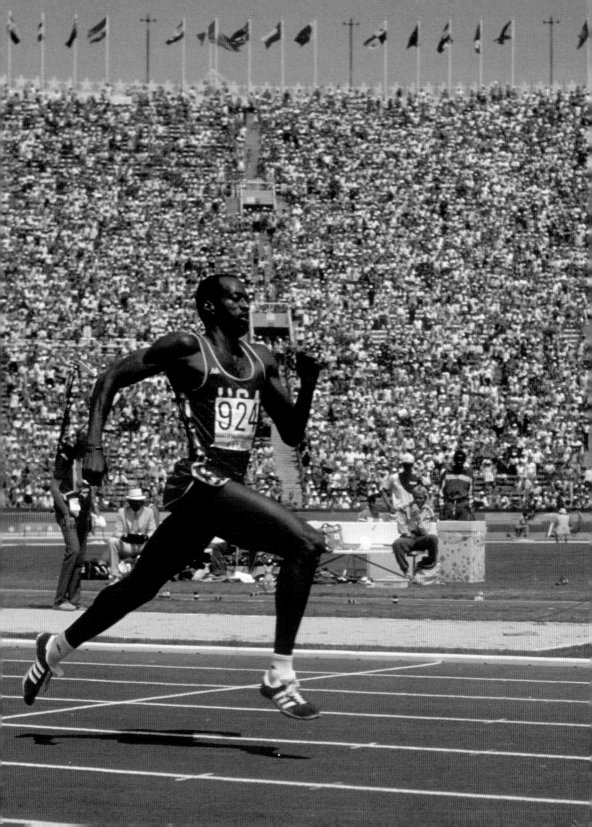

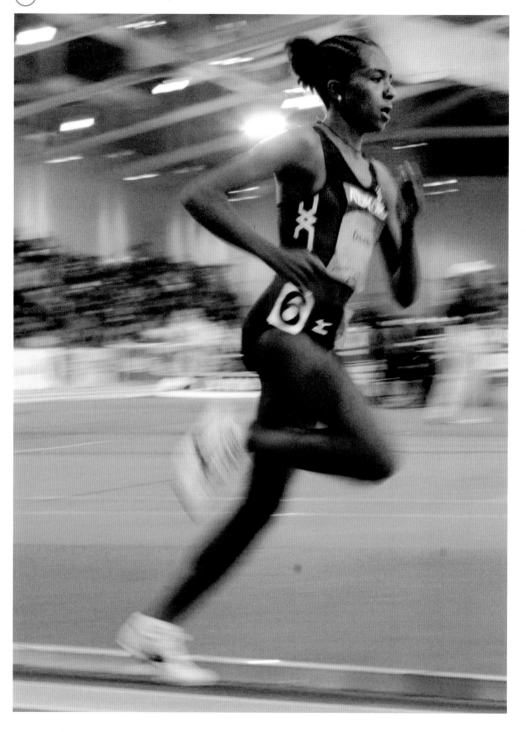

to create the next moment of support. Pose assumes that running technique is the same for all athletes, regardless of speed or distance.

Chi running, as described in a book of the same name by Danny Dreyer, has many elements in common with Pose and also emphasizes the importance of using gravity rather than muscle power as the primary source of propulsion. See the reference section for more information on both these approaches.

Implication for runners: *these are intelligent, user-friendly running approaches which (especially in the case of Pose Method) improve the ability to maintain good use in activity.*

◀ *TIRUNESH DIBABA*

Ethiopian Tirunesh Dibaba, the first woman to achieve the 5,000 m and 10,000 m double at a world championships, showing terrific form – falling upward (keeping her length) as she falls forward.

My story: Andrew Shields

As a young sprinter and jumper, competition was for me the very essence of athletics. I considered that training had value solely as preparation for performance, while the only thing that mattered about competition was winning. And if I couldn't win, setting a personal-best time or distance was a very poor consolation. It was a classic 'end-gaining' approach.

Analysis? Virtually none (though it must be remembered that this was an era before the widespread use of video, when cameras still required film rather than megapixels). I would watch other athletes, but mainly to see how far they jumped or how quickly they ran. I never felt the need to study their preparation, to try and learn from what they did differently. I also stuck rigidly to my own techniques. Looking back, my idea of progression was to work solely within what I already knew. Which, as a 20-year-old who had reached national standard on raw talent and what would now be called cross-training, was not a lot.

The inevitable consequence was injury. Simply playing football, cricket and rugby is hardly the best conditioning for the rigours of triple jumping – and when an out-of-control leap went from hop to step to collapse, it effectively ended my competitive career. I crawled out of the jumping pit and into physiotherapy for a lumbar spine fracture.

Fast-forward twenty years. Playing other sports, coaching, the burgeoning 'gym culture' and a career writing about sport and fitness had kept me in good shape – and at forty, I decided to buy a new pair of running spikes. The challenge was partly to see how much of that youthful pace remained, but mainly to discover whether greater self-knowledge, in particular my introduction to the Alexander Technique, would allow me to run with my brain as well as my body. I accepted that trying to triple jump again would probably send me into rehab, but reasoned that sprinting and the long jump would be fine.

But with a busy job, other sporting interests, a career and a family to keep me busy, where was the time to get down to the track? I decided that

I would increase my athletics-related fitness training at the gym and aim to include some track work around my coaching commitments.

I also fitted in some sessions with Malcolm Balk. We worked on some of the routines outlined in these pages, particularly those designed to rebalance the relationship between the head, neck and spine, and to develop appropriate arm movements. I found some of my old habits returning, such as a tendency to pull my head back and compress the vertebrae in my neck, but I worked to forestall these habitual patterns. I 'remembered to remember' the importance of keeping my head and back flexible and remaining poised to choose how best to use my body.

I also made one other crucial decision: to pay almost no attention to the times I ran or the distances I jumped. I wanted to enjoy the experience of competing while leaving my juvenile obsession with success well and truly in the background. Why try and hang on to the performances of two decades ago? If I performed well, I would keep it in perspective. And if I performed badly, I would spend a few moments thinking about what went wrong but then enjoy the camaraderie of my rivals.

Masters athletics is blessed with a wonderful creation: age-graded tables. These allow you to see how your current performance corresponds to an open (age 20–30) equivalent. If, as a 45-year-old, I run 12.50 for the 100 m, that corresponds to an open equivalent of 11.53. Well, I used to run faster than that, so I know there's room for improvement. If I key in my personal best of 11.2, I discover that as a 45-year-old I should be running 12.13. Hey, that's pretty quick!

The beauty of age-graded tables is that they don't deny the ageing process, they acknowledge and respect it. And the key to my continuing in track and field is that they offer scope for working with one's self: to practise, to learn, to listen to one's body, to set realistic targets. And to take pleasure in trying to improve – which is within the power of all of us, regardless of our age.

My story: Malcolm Balk

One of the highlights of the last five years has been my decision to run a marathon after a twenty-five-year break. Being a confirmed 'end-gainer', I naturally set an 'impossible' target: 2 hrs 50 mins at the age of fifty (a time I had not managed to achieve when I was thirty). Could I – or would I – 'walk the talk'?

This launched a year of 'going back to basics'. Up to this point, my long run was a 50-min, 12-km (7½-mile) Sunday morning stroll, to work up an appetite for bacon and pancakes. Thinking back to when I first trained for a marathon, I had strong memories of fighting various injuries and bugs. Could I, armed with nearly a quarter of a century of experience as an Alexandrian runner, create a different scenario this time around: fewer injuries, fewer colds and, most importantly, a better performance (my first marathon was completed in a desultory 3 hrs 37 mins)?

Since there's nothing like experience for learning, off I went – building up my distance, increasing the length of my long run, doing all the necessary things to run a marathon successfully. This time, however, I was determined to avoid injury at all cost. From past experience, I knew that increases in training were swiftly followed by a cold or an injury, or both, so I decided to keep to less than 60 km (37 miles) per week. Having a two-year-old son made this easier than I thought, as pushing a baby jogger, no matter how light the frame or how big the wheels, is no fun!

No one was optimistic about my chances of running under 2:50 on this modest amount of training but I persevered, emphasizing quality over quantity and eliminating junk miles. This paid off, in that my half-marathon time improved to the extent that I set a personal best at the age of forty-nine. I also concentrated on form. In addition to the basic Alexander Technique directions, I incorporated some of the principles of Nicholas Romanov's Pose Method, which blended beautifully.

Did I get injured? Did I catch a cold? Yes and no. One cold over the course of a year is about par for most people. As for injuries, there were nagging aches, particularly in my feet. The difference was my ability to manage minor pains before they developed into full-blown problems. I didn't take more than three days off at a stretch over the entire year.

And so to the big day. Perfect weather: cool and sunny with a light breeze. Damn, no excuses in sight! As the race unfolded, I quickly realized that I was behind my target pace, and to make it up I was going to have to expend more effort than I thought wise at that early stage. Decision time: let go of the 2:50 goal, just focus on staying smooth and easy, and see what happens. I hit the halfway mark in just under ninety minutes and it didn't feel as easy as I would have liked.

Up to this point I had been running in Pose – that is, landing on the balls of my feet and using my hamstrings to get the feet off the ground as I fell forwards (and up). By about 25 km (15½ miles), my hamstrings were getting very tired and sore. Then a younger runner who had been shadowing me for some time decided to make his move and, as he passed, called a cheery 'Looking good, buddy.' For some reason, this really annoyed me. After inhibiting and directing, my second reaction was to say to myself, 'I'm not going to let that @##$@$@ go!' So I switched back to my old style of running, namely heel-toe. Perhaps because different muscles were being engaged, I found a new level of energy, and caught up then moved ahead of my friend, wishing him a silent but no less cheery 'Do I still look good, mate?' So much for the Zen of running!

My plan was to accelerate with 5 km (3 miles) remaining and finish in style. As I approached this point, I went back to Pose and was pleased to find that my hamstrings had recovered. My pace quickened and I sped along, beginning to enjoy the race again. As I got close to the finish, someone yelled encouragingly: 'Go for it, you can still break three hours.' I had given up on a specific time and just wanted to finish – but on hearing these words I found another gear and sneaked under the three-hour barrier with seconds to spare.

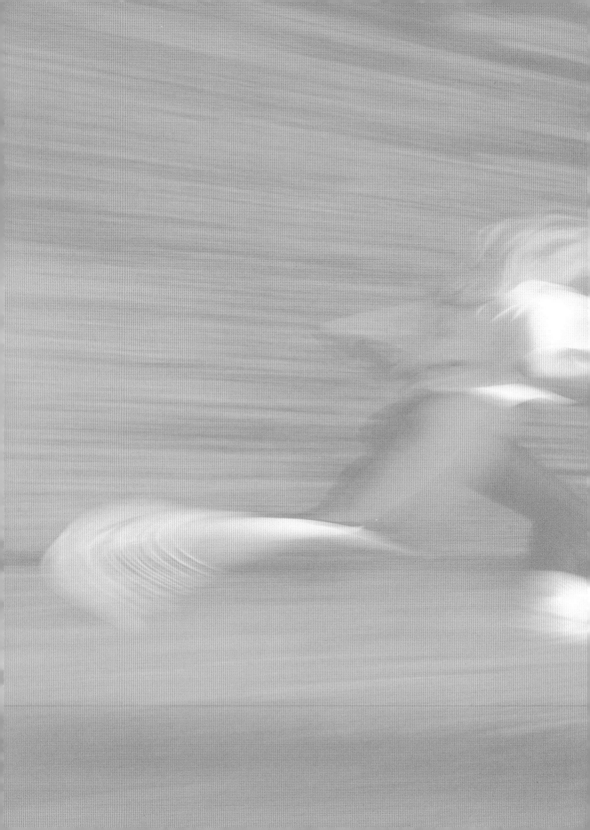

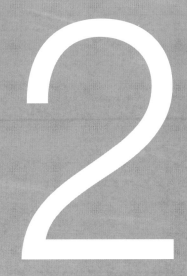

DEVELOPING AWARENESS

'Physical fitness is not only one of the most important keys to a healthy body, it is the basis of dynamic and creative intellectual activity.' **John F. Kennedy**

Australia is one of the world's most sporty and health-loving nations, from its famous cricket and rugby teams to the swimmers and surfers who relish the superb climate and outdoor lifestyle. It has produced legendary athletes such as Herb Elliott, Ron Clarke and Cathy Freeman, while generations of its top exercise professionals and sports scientists have propelled the fitness industry forward.

However, those involved in all this activity may be less familiar with another Australian, called Frederick Alexander. They may wonder what an actor whose early career was plagued by chronic hoarseness and laryngitis might have to offer top-class runners, or how his discoveries could influence the philosophy of leading coaches and fitness experts.

Who was Alexander?

Frederick Matthias Alexander (1869–1955) specialized in dramatic and humorous monologues. His story reflects a feeling that many runners, gym regulars and sports players may have had at one time or another: 'I know I can do better, so why isn't it happening for me? I have all this potential but I don't know how to realize it.' Alexander loved to perform and recite, but he suffered from a problem that prevented him doing so to the best of his ability. On stage, he would go hoarse and have to cut short his performance.

Unlike his material, this was no laughing matter. So Alexander did what most of us would have done under the circumstances: he sought advice from the medical profession, none of which was very helpful except the suggestion that he should rest. However, as soon as he put his voice to the test again, the hoarseness would recur.

Finally, he decided to tackle the problem himself. He reasoned that there must be a link between the way he recited and the difficulty with his voice. To find out what was happening, he set up mirrors so he could observe himself while speaking. He immediately noticed several habits that seemed worth investigating: there was an increased tension in his throat, his breathing and his neck as he began to recite. Further observation showed that these changes occurred not just when he spoke, but from the moment he started to think about speaking. 'I saw that as soon as I started to recite, I tended to pull back the head, depress the larynx and suck in breath through the mouth in such a way as to produce a gasping sound,' he later wrote. He realized that his problem could not be seen as merely physical, but involved his physical, mental and emotional make-up. In other words, his entire being was implicated.

Alexander began to explore different ways to release these tensions. Through experiments, he discovered that there was a strong interconnection between his head, neck and back – which he called 'the primary control of use'. Any interference with this relationship seemed to have an indirect effect not only on his voice but on his overall functioning. He also realized that there was an important link between what, and how, he was thinking, and what he found himself actually doing. If he tried to correct what he observed in the mirror, for example by putting his head in a 'better position', the results were short-lived. In order to make a reliable and long-lasting change, he realized that first and foremost, he had to prevent the wrong response from occurring. Mastering this skill enabled Alexander to perform without injury as well as to enjoy an improvement in his overall health.

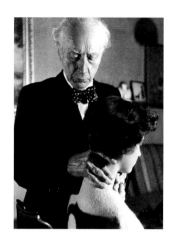

Frederick Matthias Alexander (1869–1955)

Upon returning to the stage, he encountered other actors with similar problems to his own. He offered them advice and hands-on help, and they improved as well. He moved to London in 1904 and developed his technique as a way of becoming aware of and preventing the unnecessary tension we put into everything we do, in order to function in a more free and natural fashion. Henry Irving, Lillie Langtry and Herbert Beerbohm Tree were among the many actors who later studied his methods, which became known as the Alexander Technique. Alexander continued to take on pupils – he never called them patients – including Aldous Huxley, Adrian Boult and George Bernard Shaw, the last of that trio starting lessons when he was eighty. John Cleese, Paul Newman, Maggie Smith, Paul McCartney, Daley Thompson, Linford Christie and John McEnroe are more recent pupils, while the Technique is part of the curriculum at institutions ranging from the Royal Academy of the Dramatic Arts (RADA) to the American Conservatory Theatre, San Francisco.

Alexander's discoveries

Alexander was neither an athlete nor a fitness buff. However he could, in today's terms, be described as a master personal trainer. He was concerned with the 'use of the self' – a concept that emphasizes as its core message, more than any other method around then or since, the primary significance of unity of mind and body in every act we perform. To quote Sir Charles Sherrington, the 1932 Nobel Prize winner in physiology and medicine: 'Each waking day is a stage dominated for good or ill, in comedy, farce or tragedy, by a dramatis persona – the self. And so it will be until the final curtain drops. The self is a unity.' This has universal applications for our health and well-being. However, Alexander did not start out with such grandiose ambitions but, as we have seen, simply wanted to find a way to project his voice on stage without going hoarse.

From our perspective, Alexander's realization of use is extremely valuable for anyone trying to improve or maintain their fitness. 'Being in shape' is about more than how much you weigh, how long you can run for, the size of your biceps or the poundage on your bench-press bar. The way you 'use yourself' determines the way you function. For example, if you regularly visit the gym and exercise to improve your posture but spend the rest of the day slumped in front of a computer and television, which of those actions is going to have the greater effect? And, to take the point even further, how much improvement can you expect to make if your slumping habit permeates every exercise you perform to 'correct' it?

The many hours Alexander spent observing himself in his quest to change the well-entrenched psychophysical pattern that threatened to end his acting career proved beyond a doubt that trying to overpower a bad habit by immediate and direct means doesn't work. What we resist persists! In other words, if you use yourself poorly while you exercise, you run the grave risk of reinforcing what you are already doing badly: practice, after all, makes permanent. To change functioning you first need to change use, and not the other way round.

Primary control of use

Alexander found that his vocal difficulties were related to a general pattern of interference with the natural relationship between his head, neck and back. He realized that this was the key area to focus on when 'unlearning' habitual reactions and tensions. This area exerts a powerful influence on the way we function (including, of course, the way we walk, run, lift, stand and sit). Ideally, the neck should be free of unnecessary tension – that is, not pulling the head down into the spine. The head should be poised freely on top of the spine in such a way that the spine is encouraged to lengthen and the back to widen. This produces ease, effortlessness and a sense of lightness in movement.

The difference between this state and what is usually called 'good posture' is that the latter is achieved only by fixing and holding in place various parts of the body. It's characterized by exhortations such as 'Tighten your abs' and 'Squeeze your bottom.' These direct instructions are designed to get an instant result.

Another key element in Alexander's concept of good use is what he called 'quickening the mind'. It is a state of receptivity in which we are simultaneously aware of both what we are doing and how we are doing it. For example, a good driver will notice what is not happening (tailgating, speeding, leaving the indicator on, rubbernecking and so on) as well as what is (foot on the accelerator, hands on the steering wheel, proximity of other cars).

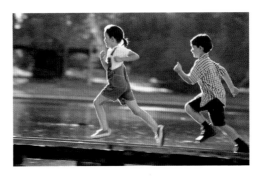

Children usually provide good examples of free and undistorted movement. These two are giving an excellent demonstration of 'natural running'.

Some of us, however, have a limited awareness of what we are doing. Whatever the activity we are engaged in, there is far more going on than we think or feel we are doing. We may habitually sit chatting to friends with our legs crossed and simply not notice that our lower back has collapsed backwards and our breathing has been compromised. We may pick up a drink and not observe that we jut our chin forwards and sharply retract our head as our lips reach the glass – a habit that can, with time, create a humped back. We are not aware of these 'extra' things we are doing when we are interested in other matters like talking or drinking. It is even possible to try hard to stand up straight and tall, but actually be more hollow-backed (that is, not straight) and shorter (by stiffening) than our real height – the opposite of what we feel we are doing. This is 'faulty sensory awareness', and we will find out more about it in Chapter 3. Eliminating these extra actions, which are are wasteful of our energy and power, is one of the most important factors in changing our way of doing anything.

Recognition of the force of habit

For so many of us, running tends to follow a familiar routine. If it's Monday, it must be an easy 5 km (3 miles). Wednesday, brisk running for thirty minutes. Friday, the 4-km (2½-mile) route you measured out in the car. Sunday, the hour with your friend that always seems to finish at a bar, with an equally long 'recovery' period spent drinking.

Following a routine is not bad. Besides, the challenge of continually coming up with new training ideas is not easy. The problem is how to prevent the familiar from becoming mechanical, where the predictability of a routine dulls the brain and you are no longer so aware of what you're doing.

This lack of connection with what is happening in the moment has many consequences. The obvious one is boredom, but it can also have an impact on achievement. In one study, a woman using a treadmill became so engrossed in listening to music that thirty minutes' work seemed like five minutes' work. The problem here was that she only seemed to derive five minutes of benefit from it, no doubt because her focus was on the music and not on the effort she was expending – or, more probably, not expending – on the treadmill. After several months, her level of fitness had shown little improvement. The solution was to get her to leave the iPod at home and simply run, so that thirty minutes actually felt like thirty minutes. When this happened, she began to make positive gains.

A different study looked at the advantages and disadvantages of running when 'associated' (switched on) and 'disassociated' (switched off). People who disassociate tend to distract themselves from discomfort, pain or tedium by thinking of something more pleasant – for example, a warm beach (let's be honest, how many of us, when sloshing through the icy winter rain, have not imagined ourselves relaxing in the sunshine, catching a few rays?). But runners who associate, the research showed, pay more attention to the signals coming from their muscles and joints and use this information to release build-ups of tension. In the study, the latter group performed better. This suggests that runners benefit from paying attention and relaying accurate information to the brain.

There are other disadvantages to what Professor Frank Pierce Jones, one of the first teachers to conduct scientific research on the Alexander Technique, called 'automatic performance'. The chief of these is that without awareness, things cannot be changed. Socrates, when asked whether it was better to do wrong knowingly or unknowingly, shocked his listeners by replying that it was better to do wrong knowingly. If you know that doing something is wrong, he explained, you can change.

It's important to mention that there is a difference between habits that are developed consciously and those that sneak in when you aren't paying attention. To use a car/driver analogy, you probably learned to drive by following a series of steps, such as getting in, putting on the seat belt, putting the key in the ignition, and so on. With experience, you can follow these steps in a state close to unconsciousness, as many of us do when setting off for work early in the morning. But, and this is the difference, if you ever found yourself in an unfamiliar make of car, you could, by reviewing the basics, probably figure out how to drive it. If you never went through the process of learning the basics, it would be more difficult.

Consciously learned habits are easier to recall and therefore to change.

When it comes to the ways in which we generally conduct ourselves, it is safe to assume that most were not learned consciously. Unless we are in pain or recovering from an injury, we don't think about how we walk, stand or lift something. As the Nike ad says, we 'just do it'. In our culture, these patterns – which we might call 'default programs' – gradually deteriorate. Just observe the default mode for sitting at the computer or in front of the television. Are we unconsciously reinforcing our 'default programs' when we run?

Inhibition

'Inhibition' is a decision not to react immediately to a stimulus. As we are constantly bombarded with stimuli, it takes awareness and practice to notice what our immediate reactions to them are. For example, a stranger walks up to you, holding out a hat. You stiffen and ready yourself to reject his plea for small change, only to realize that he is returning the headgear you have absent-mindedly left on a park bench. Or someone overtakes us in a race and we tighten and lunge in an effort to catch them.

Untying our responses from the stimuli that provoke them can open up all kinds of possibilities. Learning to inhibit the old, unwanted response permits a new response to occur unimpeded, which can then be cultivated and explored. Furthermore, inhibition is a skill we need to survive in everyday life: remembering to pause and look both ways before crossing the road can do much to prolong a running career! The challenge is remembering to remember.

Alexander used the word 'inhibition' to mean the recognition of poor use and habitual reactions, and the ability to consciously prevent or 'inhibit' them. Here's an example of inhibition in action:

A middle-distance runner decided to give the marathon a try. A friend offered him the following advice: 'The first time you feel like going [that is, increasing your pace], don't! The second time you feel like going, do not!! The third time you feel like going, if you still have something left, go!!!' By inhibiting his natural instinct to increase his pace, running with his brain in gear as well as his body , the runner recorded a time five minutes faster than his objective, finishing in a very respectable 2 hrs 31 mins.

Alexander originally developed the skill of inhibition to help him change a pattern that was threatening his career. He had to relearn how to recite without putting so much strain on his vocal apparatus that it would fail him when he

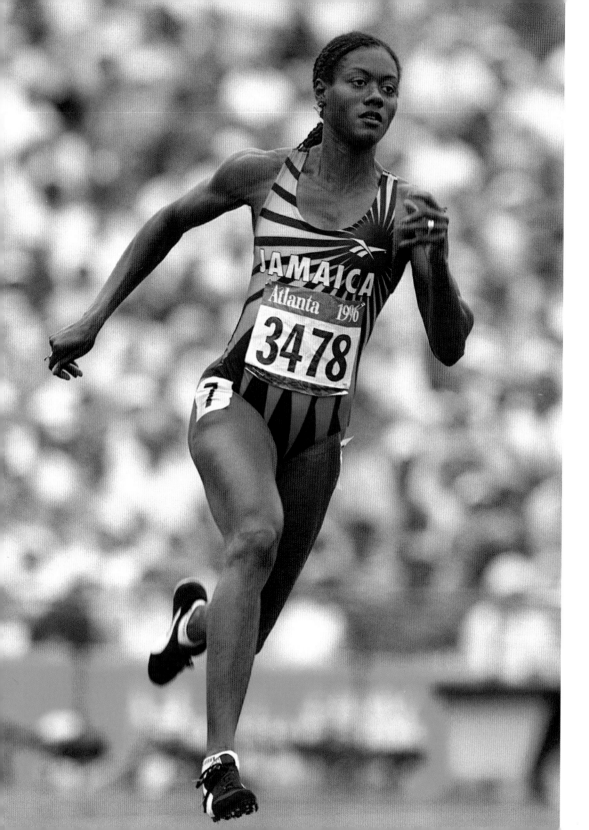

needed it most – when he was on stage, trying to entertain. Inhibition was the key that eventually enabled him to improve not only his voice, but his overall health.

Simply put, inhibition is a matter of taking advantage of the space between stimulus and response, between when you decide to do something and the moment you put that decision into action. For runners, we could formalize this as follows:

Stimulus: to increase speed.
Pause (inhibition): prevent tendency to contract back of the neck, push head forwards, and so on.
Response: increase arm rhythm.

A simple challenge is to pause before standing up, even if it's only for one second. When I asked my pupils to do this, they reported that they habitually got up and were halfway out of the room before they remembered the instruction, if they remembered at all. Likewise, it can be tough getting sprinters to pause before tackling accelerations, so they have time to review certain technical demands. By the time they're running, it's too late: they have to pause and think (or 'direct', in Alexander's words) before they act. As Alexander found when reciting, the mere idea is enough to cause a habitual reaction.

Non-doing

This term certainly does not mean doing nothing! To understand 'non-doing', let's begin with the concept of 'doing'. This means using muscles in such a way that you use more effort than the task requires, such as gripping a pencil with the force needed to swing an axe. In the Alexander context, doing implies some sort of interference with the head, neck and back relationship. While we often think of doing in terms of excessive muscular tension, it can also manifest as insufficient muscular engagement, or a lack of tone. In a non-doing approach, the emphasis is on using muscles at their maximum length at all times. So contracting is not emphasized and releasing is. When approaching a task such as lifting a weight, instead of anticipating the effort required, consider how much release you can employ to minimize the over-tensioning of muscles. Use the whole body in the action rather than just a small group of muscles. Non-doing involves the

◀ *MERLENE OTTEY*
Demonstrating the secret of her longevity as a world-class sprinter: 'effortless effort'. Here, Ottey manages to combine efficiency and grace with immense power.

skill of moving without strain: allowing, rather than imposing. Many of the world's great sportspeople and dancers, and most small children, provide excellent examples of non-doing in action. Hence the idea of 'less is more' – so long as it's the right kind of less!

That said, non-doing is difficult for us to grasp, because Western culture places so much value on doing and on progress. Even our leisure tends to be busy and mindless. The joy of non-doing is that nothing else needs to happen for this moment to be complete. The great American writer Thoreau said: 'It was morning, and lo, now it is evening, and nothing memorable is accomplished.' For go-getting, progress-oriented people, this is like waving a red flag in front of a bull. But who is to say that this has less merit than a lifetime of 'busyness', lived with scant appreciation for stillness and the present moment?

End-gaining

'End-gaining' is the plague of time-challenged modern life. It's the habit of working directly and immediately for goals and results at any cost. We all end-gain, with our hasty, over-energetic reactions to targets, which we feel we must reach as quickly as possible so that we can move on to the next one. Crossing the street before the traffic lights change, we get caught in the middle, with cars whizzing by on either side. Late for an appointment, we guess at the route to take and end up getting lost. In a hurry to get on with a workout, we yank two heavy dumb-bells from the rack and injure a shoulder.

Any gym provides a perfect illustration of end-gaining: it's full of people in a hurry to get their workout over and move on to the rest of the day. Not everyone is there for the intrinsic pleasure and challenge of exercising safely and effectively, but for such extrinsic motivations as pleasing a partner or doing what the doctor suggested. A lack of enjoyment is manifest in the speed at which people complete their routine and their lack of attention to it. As for good form – forget it. Equipment manufacturers collude in this process with the book rack on the exercise bike and the holder for the personal stereo on the treadmill. Then there's the 'cardio theatre', with ranks of exercise machines arranged in front of TV and video screens that offer distractions to overcome 'the boredom of training', and which further diminish the process.

When it comes to competitive running, end-gaining is almost ubiquitous. Let's look at a common example: the speed you run at. Form is sacrificed for speed, with the result that potential is soon limited by poor technique. It's called 'running with the brakes on'. I worked with a runner who was suffering from this problem. I asked Peter, a 28-year-old runner (5 km/3 miles in 21 mins), to run beside me so I could give him some feedback while he was in motion. By the time I had reached the hypothetical starting line, he was 15 m (49 ft) in front of me. Several attempts to rein him in all ended in failure. On paper, I was a much faster runner. So why was he unable to humour me at my pedestrian pace? Runners, like amateur musicians, tend to rush – perhaps under the misguided notion that this will make them faster. It does, up to a point – and then they get stuck. In Peter's case, judging from his physique and ability to sprint, he was certainly capable of running much faster than his 5-km 'personal best' would indicate. So what was his problem? Peter was a one-gear runner. And, even worse, he didn't know it. His gear, way too fast for an easy jog, was way too slow when it came to recording a 5-km (3-mile) time nearer to his potential.

There are several ways to deal with this situation. One is to practise running with control – very slowly, with good use and excellent form. It is possible to run at a pace of 12 mins per 1.6 km (1 mile), maintaining good form and taking 180 strides per minute. However, most runners' form goes right down the pan when they run as slowly as this. Try it for yourself.

The other advantage of running slowly is that you will notice more about your running style: light or heavy footfall, swaying, time on the ground, unnecessary tension, head movement and so on – most of which you willl be oblivious to at faster tempos.

Run with a friend who has an easy pace that is slower than yours, and match it. Make it a game in which every time you go ahead of her it'll cost you an ice cream or a beer.

Practise training at specific speeds. For those of you who like to run intervals on the track and enjoy a bit of maths, Frank Horwill (coach, writer, raconteur and founder of the British Milers' Club) created a five-tier training system which was adopted by Peter Coe when he coached his son Sebastian to double Olympic gold in the 1980s. Horwill's theory was that we need to train our ability to run at different speeds or paces, from 800 m to the marathon. He calculated that the difference between each level (800 m, 1,500 m, 3,000 m, 5,000 m and 10,000 m) was four seconds (five seconds for women). So, let's say that you can run 10 km (6 miles) in 40 mins. This works out at 4 mins per km, or 1 min 36 secs for 400 m (one lap). Therefore, your potential time for 5 km (3 miles) would be 1 min 32 secs per lap, giving a time of 19 mins 16 secs. A 3-km (2-mile) pace is 4 secs faster at

1 min 28 secs per lap, giving you a potential time of 11 mins. To run 1,500 m would take 1 min 24 secs per lap – giving a time of 5 mins 15 secs. For 800 m it would be 1 min 20 secs per lap, giving a time of 2 mins 40 secs for the distance.

Runners should tackle practice sessions at these various paces. A sample training session at an 800-m pace for our 40-min, 10-km (6 mile) runner would be 8 x 400 m in 1 min 20 secs with a 3-min jog recovery between each repetition. By training at different tempi, you will develop better pace judgement as well as the discipline to tame your tendency to run either too slowly or too fast. Then you can choose the speed at which you run more effectively, instead of staying stuck in the same old gear. See Frank Horwill's excellent book, *Obsession for Running*, for more on this approach.

The means whereby

An 'end-gaining' approach is judged mostly on outcomes: the amount of weight on the bar, the length of time on the treadmill, the number of kilos lost in a month, and so on. While it is useful to have objective ways of measuring progress, the outcome of any activity is just an indicator of progress. If it is relied on as the only indicator, this can result either in a false sense of accomplishment or a feeling of failure if the expected targets are not met. Albert Einstein captured the essential futility of this approach when he stated: 'Not everything that counts can be counted and not everything that can be counted counts.'

Competitive people often judge success by end-gaining standards. However, competitiveness is not a requirement for maintaining or improving fitness. It may well, in fact, make it more difficult to do so. Real progress is more often achieved when competitive urges are mitigated by a greater concentration on the process of an activity – this is known as the 'means whereby'.

Here's an illustration. It's indisputable that a half-hour run, three or four times a week, will bring significant health benefits, particularly in terms of cardiovascular efficiency. However, it's all too easy to move from being a 'fun' runner, where the activity is enjoyed for its own sake, to the more serious version where times, distances and race results become the *raison d'être* of the sport. Miss a day? Run a poor time? You've failed! Add on injuries, fatigue and mood change (such as excessive grumpiness after the aforementioned poor time), and running becomes another stick with which to beat yourself.

How can Alexander's discoveries help runners?

If Alexander had been a runner rather than an actor, what would his story have been? Perhaps something like this. Our young Australian (let's call him FM) was very promising over 800 m. He enjoyed early success and achieved a national ranking, but was soon plagued by injuries that threatened his career. Medical attention and a constant supply of gimmicky new shoes provided only short-term relief, because as soon as he resumed serious training, he injured himself once again and was forced back into the tedious process of rest and rehabilitation.

When doctors proposed risky surgery as the only solution, FM decided to take matters into his own hands. He reasoned that there must be something in the way he ran that was causing his problems, since he only injured himself when he trained and raced. Setting up a video camera, he filmed himself from several angles. On viewing the results, he noticed several things that his track pals had often joked about. When he ran, he tended to pull his head back, breathe in loudly through his mouth, tighten and arch his lower back, and pound his feet on the ground. His friends told him that these habits were more pronounced at the finish of a race, when he looked like someone who was being attacked by a swarm of bees. Further study revealed that many of these running habits were also present when he walked, though they were less noticeable.

Through constant observation and experimentation, FM found that if he could maintain the poise of his head on top of his spine when he ran, this had a positive influence on the rest of his body patterns: he stopped gasping for air, arching and stiffening his back, and the ground no longer echoed to the pounding of his feet.

However, maintaining these improvements when he ran, and particularly when he raced, proved more difficult. He noticed that in moments of pressure or stress, he would usually revert to his old habits. What, then, are the benefits for FM in learning and applying some of Alexander's principles?

Developing fitness and form

The late George Sheehan, doctor, runner, writer and philosopher, wrote this when in his seventies: 'One way I have aged is in my appearance and in the way I go about normal activities. Carriage is important – and mine is poor. Having good posture, flexibility and a spring in your step makes for a youthful impression. But I have poor flexibility, terrible posture, and tend to stroll rather than stride. If you saw me walking around town, you would think I was older than I am. *This form of ageing is, of course, completely unnecessary* [my italics].'

THE BENEFITS OF LEARNING ALEXANDER'S PRINCIPLES

Universality

Alexander's principles can be applied anywhere, any time. They require no special equipment or help. They can and should be used before, during and after running.

Autonomy

Like a language, once you learn the principles and how to apply them, you can benefit from them. They are yours to do with as you wish.

Causes of problems

The principles deal with causes, not just symptoms. They can help in many other areas of life as part of a generalized, ongoing process of improvement.

Balance and coordination

Improvements in balance and coordination lead to more efficient movement with less wasted effort. Energy can be directed to where it will give the greatest return.

Injury prevention

Being receptive to feedback and signals from the body enables a runner to ease off before a niggle becomes a nightmare.

Choice

There are many different ways of running: fast, slow, uphill or down, into the wind, on different surfaces, barefoot or shod, in hot or cold weather, at various altitudes, straight, zigzagging, alone or in a pack, on the track, on the beach. Good runners adapt their running form in order to meet each condition effectively. This might mean lengthening or shortening the stride, more or less use of the arms, changing the amount of forward lean, altering the amount of knee or heel lift, landing more towards the heel or more towards the ball of the foot, varying breathing rhythms, and so on.

Poor running form, coupled with lack of awareness of oneself and one's environment, leads to statements like: 'I can't run fast when it's cold.' Choosing not to run outside when its -1°C and you are worried about frostbite can be a wise decision, but not running outside at all in the winter because you don't know how to do it safely is denying yourself a potentially wonderful experience. Improving overall balance, coordination and awareness gives the runner more tools to employ and makes it far easier to adapt to different circumstances.

Often, in trying to reach our goals, we sacrifice form for fitness. This is a mistake and results in unnecessary stress and strain, which ultimately works against the original intention. This notion takes me back to my days as an ice hockey player. In my innocent arrogance, I believed that my abilities and success were clear indications of my highly developed coordination and evolution as a human being. The fact that my 'form' was really pathetic the moment I left the ice was of little concern to me. In fact, I used to revel in my version of cat-like repose.

It was only when my superior beliefs about my coordination were put to the test, as I tried to apply my habitual approach to playing the cello, that I began to suspect that all was not as wonderful as I had believed. At the cello, I was stiff and this decreased my ability to learn. It was only when I began taking Alexander Technique lessons that the blinkers really came off. I was increasingly aware of my tendency to slump and collapse (like many athletes, dancers, musicians and gym buffs who stop 'thinking' once they finish performing). It was as if I was disconnecting from my body.

Another area that came under scrutiny was my tendency, when things weren't going well, to force, to push, to seek a 'bigger hammer'. Looking back, it is funny how this attitude did not simply manifest itself physically but was present in all areas of life.

The basic message to learn from all this is that if a runner sacrifices form for fitness, trouble is usually not far off. Training when injured or sick is an example of putting fitness before form (that is, failing to use common sense and ignoring the far more important matter of health).

Recuperation and regeneration

For committed runners, hard work is unavoidable. However, training breaks the body down and makes it weaker. It's rest that makes the body stronger. This is known as the 'training effect', where the body adapts to the loading of the cardiovascular and muscular systems by improving the heart's efficiency, increasing the size of capillaries in the muscles and boosting glycogen and enzymes in the muscle cells. During periods of recovery, these systems build to greater levels in order to compensate for the stress that you've applied, taking your body on to a higher level of performance. Understanding the training effect means knowing how and when to stop is as important as knowing how and when to train.

Countless runners have lost the benefits of a training programme by not giving themselves time to recover, and risking the dangers of over-training or burn-out. Even elite runners should have at least one day a week of complete rest, though it can be very difficult to persuade highly motivated athletes (super end-gainers) that less training will actually mean more in terms of fitness, overall health and well-being. Instead, 'active rest' is an extremely effective means of recuperation. Rather than collapsing in front of the TV, a runner can use active rest procedures to release any unnecessary tension and re-establish a state of balanced coordination which will go a long way towards helping him reap the benefits of the training regime (see Chapter 5 for an intelligent approach to training and active rest).

Improvement

Most people who take up running never learn to run well. Sad but true, though this is not just the case for runners – the merest glance at your local tennis court, golf course or football pitch will give you plenty of examples of people playing poorly. Leaving aside the facts that physical activity should be encouraged and that people can still enjoy sports regardless of their level of skill, there are three main reasons why people perform poorly. The first is a reluctance to practise and seek guidance from qualified, experienced coaches – this is the case for most non-elite adults across every sport. The other two are, as discussed above, end-gaining and faulty sensory awareness. It's sometimes said that 90 per cent of runners are confirmed end-gainers while the other 10 per cent are confirmed liars!

While goals can provide an important source of motivation, if you focus on them too early, it can be counterproductive. Runners, especially early in their careers, are vulnerable to developing bad habits of form which will plague them for their entire running lives. It takes time to learn to run well, and that timescale can't be reduced without making serious compromises. For a person of average coordination seeking to run competitively, that may mean around five years' training.

I once worked with a runner who 'ran heavy'. You could really hear him coming. But when he applied Alexander's principles, such as maintaining his intention through inhibition (noticing when his mind wandered and refocusing) and direction (reminding himself to look ahead), he could modify his step and run much more lightly. The only problem was that he kept forgetting to pay attention and would quickly lapse into his old pattern of pounding. Finally, after I had brought his attention back to this habit once again, he exclaimed in exasperation, 'How bloody

CASE STUDY
A runner's experience: Sam

Running with my brain in gear: for me, that means a constant dialogue between my brain and body, and constant adjustment/response. Although I can still switch off – and escape stress – through running, it is more because of the distraction that running gives me rather than the idea that I am running on autopilot.

In fact, far from being on autopilot, I am actually steering the plane (my body) constantly. Does it feel better if I relax my ankles? Are my arms crossing my body a little because my shoulders are hunched? What if I pick up my feet a little? Every run is an exploration of what works and what doesn't – and it can be different every time. That's why I can't fathom why people say running is boring. How can it be boring when there is so much to learn, so much to pay attention to?

In a recent race, in which I blew my half-marathon personal-best time out of the water, I noticed that I was saying to myself: 'OK, we can sustain this pace' and 'We're doing brilliantly'. We?! It was my brain and body that I was seeing as a team. They (we!) had to work together to succeed, whether that was about going faster, winning or simply completing a tough challenge.

I have used the same strategy when coming back from injury – the idea that we must work together, body and mind, to get it right.

often do I have think about my bloody feet landing?' And of course the answer was: 'Every bloody step!'

Learning to pay attention can be difficult, but it is far from impossible. Let's return once more to the analogy with the car: when you learn to drive, at first you have to think about putting the key in the ignition, turning the engine on, and so forth. Once you become more familiar with the basics, you don't have to think about them so actively – but at the same time, in order to move the vehicle, you can't leave any of them out. Learning to 'think in activity' is essential for improvement.

Enjoyment

Everyone should take pleasure in performing the art of running well, regardless of what that means in practice. It might be running slowly, yet elegantly, through a local park. It might be floating rather than pounding on the treadmill at the gym, your body staying quiet and poised as your arms move rhythmically in sync with your legs. It might be discovering that extra gear on the home stretch and maintaining your form to the finish line. Or climbing a long hill with effortless ease, your body finding the perfect angle as you lean gently into the slope, your knees popping up with every stride and your arm movement helping to keep you light and tall over the crest of the hill. The runner who is willing to practise the art of running will experience many such moments.

HAILE GEBRSELASSIE ▶

Smiling on his way to Olympic gold in Sydney: what use, what an athlete! Gebrselassie's poise, awareness, attention to form and economy of style have confirmed his reputation as one of the all-time greats.

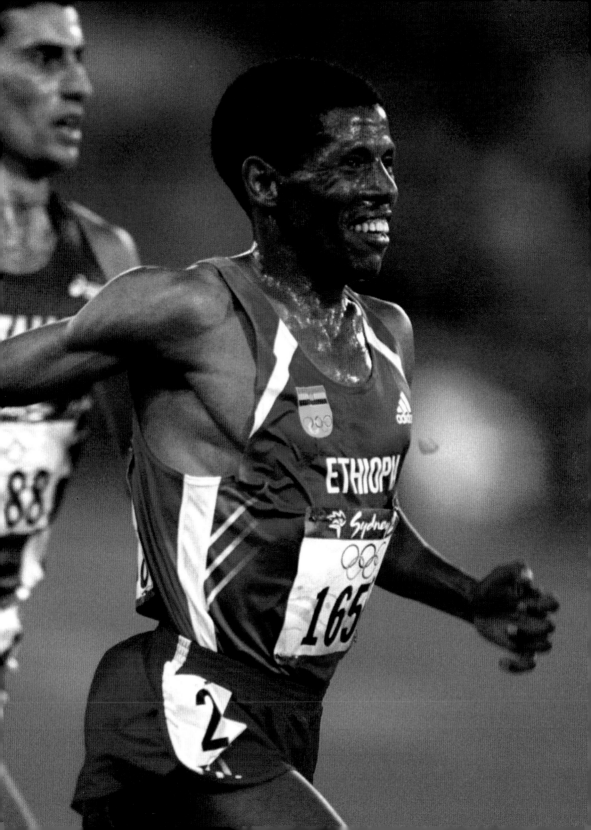

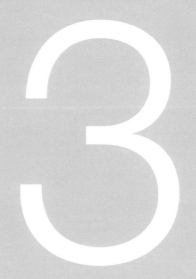

THINKING INTO MOVEMENT

'Fitness has to be fun. If it is not play, there will be no fitness.
Play, you see, is the process. Fitness is merely the product.'

Dr George Sheehan

As we have seen, the way we use ourselves affects the way we function. Acts can be performed in a number of ways, some of which are less harmful than others. Let's go back to our mechanical metaphor to make the point clear. As a runner, you are both car and driver. You only get one vehicle in this life, and in spite of advances in replacement technology (new hips, knee reconstructions), the original parts generally work best. So if you wear out the engine, strip the tyres, fry the brakes and stain the upholstery, you can't trade it in for a new model. As driving instructors everywhere will tell you, we all bring attitudes, skills and habits to bear on our car, which affect the way it performs on the road. We pop the clutch, slam on the brakes, over-rev the engine, reverse into bollards and fail to look in the mirror before changing lanes. All these factors contribute to the functioning of the vehicle and, ultimately, to the quality of the ride.

Remember the description of the 'primary control of use' in Chapter 2? This is the state achieved when the neck is free and not pulling the head down into the spine, producing ease, effortlessness and a sense of lightness in movement. It's characterized by the head being poised freely on top of the spine, so the spine lengthens and the back widens. It also accurately illustrates what coaches describe as 'running tall'.

Alexander was particularly concerned with the role that the neck plays in our use; more specifically, with the fact that most people over-tighten this area. It's a habit that is often overlooked by runners and it can strongly influence the amount of effort exerted during any activity. Indeed, there's ample research to show the critical role played by the neck in posture. In one experiment designed to demonstrate this fact, a volunteer had a local anaesthetic injected into one side of his neck. The loss of muscle sensation and of muscle tone on the injected side produced the illusion of a pull over to that side of the body. The subject reported that he felt drawn to one side like an iron bar to a magnet. He was unable to walk with any coordination, like someone who has had too much to drink. When lying down, he felt the couch was toppling over towards the side of the injection. This was because the dominating nerves in the neck help to determine how the brain controls muscles in posture and movement.

You will recall that Alexander spent a considerable amount of time observing himself in the mirror. However, his purpose was not to check for signs of a receding hairline, but to discover why his voice seemed to disappear at a time when he needed it most – on stage. You may also remember that while he watched himself recite in the mirror, he observed that he did several peculiar things, which he surmised were related to his vocal difficulties. These included tightening his neck and lifting his chin so that his head was pulled back, depressing his larynx, and breathing in through his mouth

Right The way we use ourselves affects the way we function. 'Primary control of use' is the state achieved when the neck is free and not pulling the head down into the spine, producing ease, effortlessness and a sense of lightness in movement.

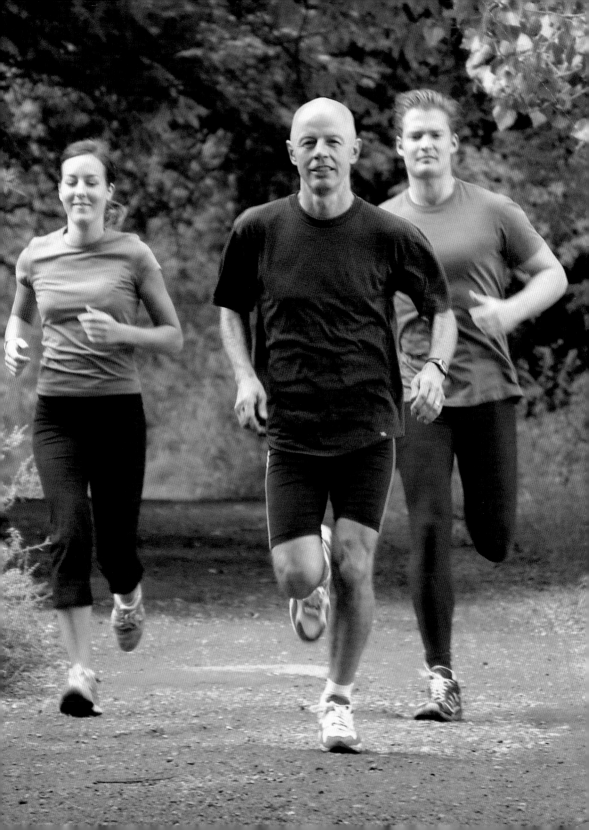

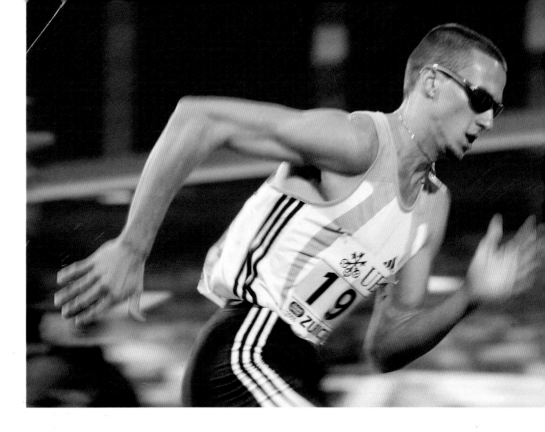

with a loud gasping sound. He subsequently noticed that he also lifted his chest, arched his back and tightened his legs and feet. Was it the sucking in of breath that caused the pulling back of the head and the depressing of the larynx?

Alexander found that he could not change his breathing or the contraction of his larynx directly, but he was able to control these harmful tendencies indirectly by preventing his head from being pulled back. Further research enabled him to see that the relationship between his head and neck also affected his torso; and for his voice to be allowed to work properly, his head had to be carried in such a way that it encouraged his back to lengthen and widen.

JEREMY WARRINER ▲

The American 400 m runner won the gold medal at the 2004 Athens Olympic Games by demonstrating the ideal combination in a competitive athlete: power, control, focus and attention to form.

Try this little experiment:

Sit on a chair, near the edge, and allow yourself to slump. Feel good? But you might notice that the back of your neck has 'disappeared' and your throat feels a little tight. Now sit up really straight, so that your chest is raised, your back is hollowed and your chin is tucked in. You may notice the same sort of feeling in your throat.

Our coordination is affected by the quality of this relationship. When we over-contract the neck and pull the head down, the spine compresses and distorts – which affects the way we use our limbs. It then takes more effort to get from A to B, and we place more strain on ourselves in the process. In other words, someone who uses herself in this way will tend to run 'a bit funny' and not make the best use of herself. It's like trying to push a rope up a hill: it can be done, but…

Vertebrate animals generally demonstrate good coordination: their head leads and their body follows. Of course, animals do not know what they are doing; they 'just do it'. We humans, on the other hand, have the mixed blessing of consciousness, which can be used to help us become more cheetah-like in our urban jungle. Nevertheless, people from less industrialized nations seem to suffer less interference with the natural use of themselves than we do in the West. For example, physiologists have found that Kenyan women use no more effort – that is, oxygen consumption – walking up a hill with a 10-kg (22-lb) jug of water balanced on their head than you or I would without one. And they haven't figured out why, as yet. (You might wonder whether if you walk around with a book on your head like the girls at charm schools used to do, you might learn to walk like a Kenyan. Try it and see!) It's likely that it's because Kenyan women already possess excellent balance and coordination. As for Kenyan men, you don't see many of them walking around with jugs

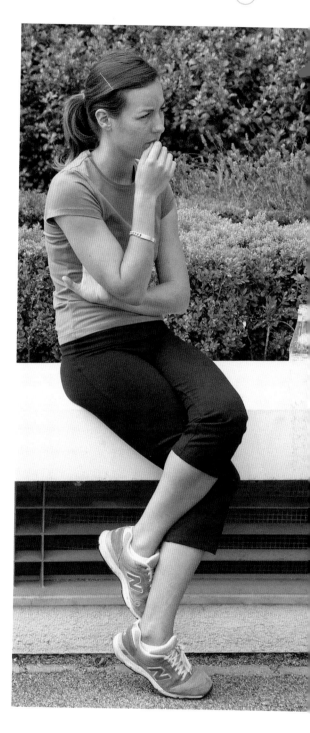

Right 'We run like we sit'. Pulling down or collapsing brings distortion of the body and a mal-distribution of effort which affect our ability to move gracefully and efficiently.

balanced on their heads, but you certainly see enough of them on the winner's rostrum at races!

Faulty sensory awareness

Ever seen yourself on video or in photographs and been surprised by what you really look like? Or have you heard your voice on an answering machine and thought that it didn't sound like you? Or have you performed a little dance move that you imagined was cool and stylish, only to be told by your best friend that you look more like an elephant on roller skates? This is called 'faulty sensory awareness'. It describes the way that we think or feel we are doing a thing when in fact we are doing something completely different. And when we try to change an ingrained habit, the new and improved version often feels odd, awkward or even wrong – which increases the likelihood of our going back to what we know, even if it isn't serving us well.

Most of us believe that if we are told (or, better still, shown) what to do, we should be able to carry out the instructions or follow the demonstration without any trouble. Sadly, reality does not support this assumption. To understand why, try this simple test:

Cross your arms. Have a look at them; notice which one is over and which is under. Now cross them the other way. Take your time! How does the new way feel? As natural and comfortable as the first? Probably not. How likely would you be to cross your arms this way if it was the 'correct' way to perform this movement?

What can we blame for this sad state of affairs? Let's put it down to faulty sensory awareness. We generally identify five senses: sight, smell, hearing, taste and touch. The nineteenth-century anatomist Charles Bell identified a sixth, which is commonly referred to as 'kinaesthesia' or 'proprioception'. It refers to our ability to know where one bit of our body is in relation to another.

Faulty sensory awareness is evident when we try to correct or improve ourselves in action or at rest, and our internal guidance system – the kinaesthetic sense – cannot be relied on to provide accurate feedback. Here's a hypothetical example: a woman has been doing circuit training during the off-season to improve her all-round fitness and feels that she has perfected the routines. But then the teacher tells her that her head is moving around all over the place during certain moves and she should think about keeping it more centred and under control. After getting over her initial shock at the comment, she does a little extra practice at home – just to see off what is obviously the instructor's compulsive pickiness about minor details. Returning triumphantly to the class, she demonstrates her newfound prowess, only to be told quietly afterwards that 'the head thing' seems a little worse than before. She can't believe it! But when the instructor takes the time to show her in the mirror, she is mortified when she realizes the instructor is right. How could this happen if she cannot even feel it?

Alexander offered a clue when he remarked that: 'You can't know a thing by an instrument

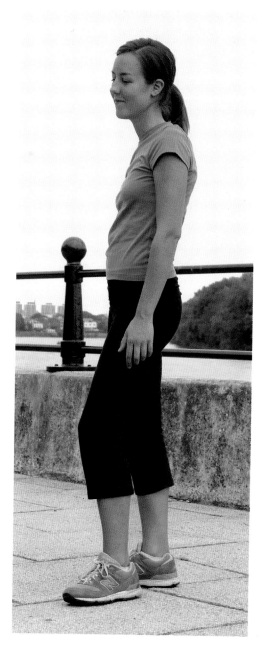

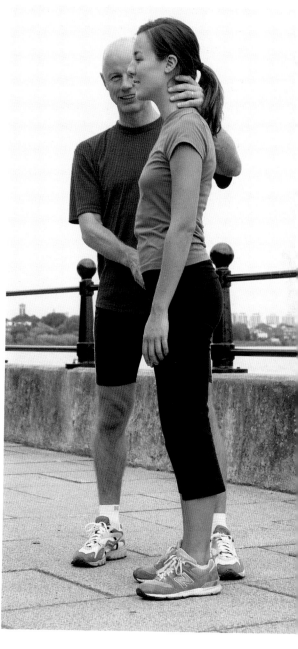

Above This runner's 'default program' when she stands tends towards a collapse, a habit which she will unfortunately bring with her when she runs.

Above Relearning to stand, with a lengthening tendency. Not only does this tidy up her profile, it will also help her move in a more integrated manner.

that is wrong.' The instrument to which he was referring is, of course, our kinaesthetic sense. The difficulty Alexander encountered, and which is widespread in today's society, is that the familiar becomes the standard by which we judge what is right and what is wrong. Since the exerciser in our scenario was trying hard to improve, we can guess with some certainty that she was doing what felt right – which was moving her head. The challenge, when trying to change an old habit, is to become comfortable with the unfamiliar. This is hard to do under the best of circumstances, but is particularly difficult when one is striving to 'get it right'.

Chronic tension also plays a role in faulty sensory awareness. Muscles that are tightened for long periods of time no longer provide the brain with feedback. In other words, we become less aware of what is going on in these areas, and it therefore becomes harder to make the decisions necessary to maintain our poise, balance and enjoyment – that is, to release unnecessary tension.

As a runner, you might recognize the following dilemma. You've just read an article on improving your running form and have decided to follow its suggestions. This decision was prompted in part by a recent picture of yourself in action looking more like a Skoda with four flat tyres than a Jaguar purring along at full throttle. And there was also that injudicious comment by a fellow athlete who said she could recognize you, even at a distance, because of the cute way you roll your shoulders and hold your head on one side – not to mention that little hitch in your stride. After several weeks of doing appropriate exercises, you believe that real progress is being made.

Much to your dismay, after videoing yourself to preserve the new you for posterity, you are shocked to see that the cute way you cock your head and roll your shoulders is still there. In fact, it seems worse! You feel upset and let down. You ask: 'How could my senses have deceived me?' Sadly, our senses do deceive us. Our kinaesthetic sense can fail to provide an accurate picture of what we are doing with ourselves – in this case the way we are running. Geoffrey Cannon describes a wonderful example of faulty sensory awareness:

I've never been the same since a run round Hyde Park and Kensington Gardens in newly fallen snow, early one winter morning four years ago. I was scheduled for three circuits: 13½ miles at a steady 8-minute-mile pace, making 1 hr 48 mins for the whole run. No big deal, I thought, and eased into the run feeling pretty pleased with myself. Nobody else was around. Or so I thought, until I reached Speakers' Corner. For there, by my side, on my own route, were a runner's footprints – and a funny sight they were, too. The prints were man-size, but the runner was taking comic little strides. What was sillier still, though, was the position of the footprints. They looked like a clock showing five minutes to two: the left foot splayed out a bit, the right foot turned some way to being back to front. A fine figure of fun he must look, I thought to myself, smugly, and carried on. Doesn't he realize how ridiculous he looks? I amused myself around

Hyde Park Corner by imitating the preposterous gait of the stumbler who, no doubt, I should soon ease past.

I never saw him, though. Instead, I was startled to see, the next time around Speakers' Corner, that there were two sets of footprints, one fairly crisp, and the other half-obscured by falling snow, right by my side, on my route. Surely there couldn't be two runners, I thought to myself. It had to be one. Odd that I hadn't caught him up. So I amused myself by running in his footprints. And then I realized. He was me. I had no idea I ran like that. For the rest of the run I tried not to believe my eyes. This must stop, I instructed myself, and made my feet parallel, and ran round in little circles to check myself out. And still the feet – my feet – were not straight. I finished the run completely deflated.

A few weeks later I could bear it no longer, and decided to have a confidential word with a compassionate runner. So I asked my co-author Alison Turnbull: 'Ali, do I ever run like this?' (deliberately exaggerating the lopsided duck's gait.) 'All the time,' she said. 'I can tell it's you 200 yards away.' And she pointed out some hilarious little ways I have with my arms when I run. I was forced to admit that, like so many runners, I had a completely inaccurate mental picture of myself in action.

Only then did I notice that the 'Permanent Record Of You To Treasure Always' photographs taken in New York's Central Park at the end of the marathon showed the real picture; as did reflective shop windows into which I started nervously glancing. Hence my

interest in movement awareness in general, and the Alexander Technique in particular.

Geoffrey Cannon, *Running Times*, November 1987

Sitting

There's a strong chance that Geoffrey Cannon runs like he sits. When I mention this in workshops, people usually react with sheepish grins and vain efforts to sit up. Runners who misuse themselves (that is, sit poorly) during their working and leisure hours are often advised to take remedial action in the form of strengthening and stretching, to counteract the self-inflicted damage.

In an article in *Sports Injury Bulletin*, physiotherapist Sean Fyfe posts a salutary reminder about the potentially adverse consequences of a sedentary day job. What is wrong with sitting? Typically, Fyfe says, sitting produces:

- Tight hip flexors, hamstrings and calves;
- Tightness through the external hip rotators, leading to restriction in hip joint range;
- Limitation of lumbar spine extension;
- Stiff thoracic spine;
- Protracted and elevated scapulae with weak lower trapezius and serratus anterior;
- Tight and weak posterior rotator cuff;
- Poked chin posture with associated weak deep neck flexors and overactive upper trapezius, levator scapula and rhomboid muscles.

Wow! That's some list! Fyfe adds, 'Prolonged sitting has also been linked to acute muscle strains in dynamic sports, in particular hamstring strains. The lumbar spine stiffness associated with sitting leads to altered neural input into the posterior thigh. This can manifest as increased muscle tone of the hamstrings, which will alter the length–tension relationship and increase the risk of strain.'

As we prepare, in our next section, to begin movement, the implications of this article are clear. Rather than just trying to fix a problem, it's essential that we learn to prevent it in the first place.

Going into movement: walking

It is possible to move in many different ways, as anyone observing a local fun run will attest. Sometimes the variations can be pretty funny, although they are usually not intended as such. It's fair to assume that you're reading this book not to develop the tragicomic aspects of your stride, but to change, reduce or eliminate them. An article by Walton L. White points out that some ways of walking (and, by extension, running) are better than others:

Some ways are basic patterns evolution worked out for us long ago; others are distortions we have imposed on these basic patterns, often with an added tax of unnecessary effort. We can become so accustomed to paying this added tax we don't recognize it as such and take it as part of the original price.

There's a big difference in the effort I make during walking when I merely extend my body upward over my foot and when I try to push the ground down and back away from me. In the first instance I just move my body away from the ground; in the second, I am trying to move the whole planet away from me. It shouldn't surprise anyone, however, that it takes more effort to push the planet than to push my body.

Walton L. White, 'Together We Walk'

The physiology of walking is resolved into the primary movements of allowing the body to incline forwards from the ankle on which the weight is supported, then to prevent oneself from falling by allowing the weight to be taken in turn by the foot that has been advanced. This method, simple as it may appear, is not how most people walk. Nearly everyone employs physical tension in such a way that there is a tendency to shorten the spine and legs, by pressing down through the floor instead of lightening that pressure by lengthening the body, throwing the weight forwards and moving lightly and freely.

The key, then, is to avoid putting the brakes on when you move – to learn how to flow, how to get out of the way and let 'it' move you. The following procedure focuses on what happens in the time between the decision to take a step and the moment when you actually take it:

Stand in front of a mirror or reflective window, with your feet fairly close together. Take a step forwards and note the amount of sway. To make this even more fun, ask a friend

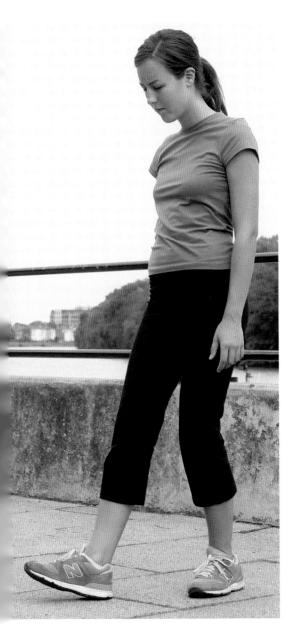

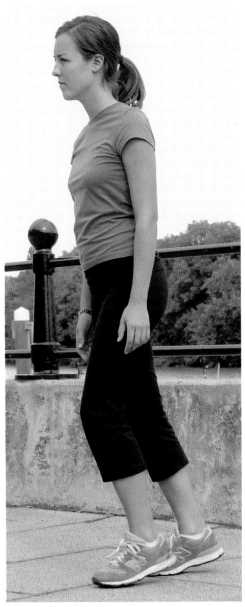

Above Going into movement the hard way – looking down by dropping the head causes heaviness, braking and requires more effort.

Above Releasing into movement. By learning how to 'fall upwards', the transition from stillness into motion becomes more of a flow than a stutter.

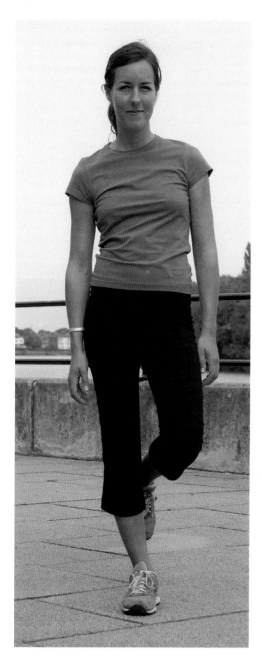 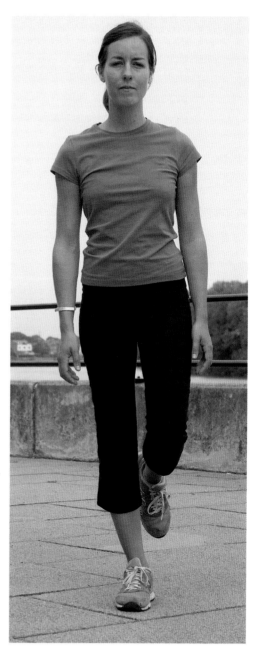

Above This is an example of an 'energy leak'. The runner's right hip has collapsed, followed by her right side and shoulder.

Above Here the runner maintains length; there are no 'leaks'. The head leads and the body follows with sufficient connection and tone to reduce waste and increase efficiency.

to watch and see if he can guess which foot you are going to step with before you actually move. Most people telegraph their intention by leaning over to one side – the left side if they are going to step with the right foot. The question that needs to be asked is why this happens and what it means for us as runners.

The act of leaning is related to our need to balance ourselves. The desire not to land on our bottom is very strong and, for the most part, unconscious. Whenever we feel out of balance, a little alarm bell goes off in the form of a 'fear reflex' and the result is that we stiffen ourselves. This is why we lean: we are simply trying not to fall over.

The significance of this for runners is that leaning from side to side is wasteful and places added stress on the side that's being leaned upon. But the good news is that it's not necessary. Just as you can learn to lift one leg off the ground and not shift everything over to the other side like an unbalanced beanbag chair, you can also learn to minimize this tendency when you run. One of the best times to learn this skill is when you go into motion.

Here is an argument overheard in a workshop as to why this is impossible: 'If I lift up my right leg, I have to shift everything over to the left. Where else is it going to go?' (This was followed by a massive lean to the left.)

And here is the clever answer: 'Rather than thinking of weight going from side to side, think of it going up and down or forwards and backwards – and maybe even both at the same time!'

There are other things to think about when taking a step. Do you tighten or release into motion – do you flow into the movement, or start things off with a little jerk? It's like learning to drive a car with a clutch. Do you want to pop it, or ease it up so that the transition from stop to start is barely perceptible? If you are properly balanced, all that it takes to move is a release in the calf muscles. Let them go and you should start to topple forwards. Pushing, shoving, leaning, reaching and stubbing are all completely unnecessary and should be eliminated. So should a heavy landing. Falling 'forward and up' will assist you in the latter. Practise a smooth move into motion whenever you can.

Here's another clever question: what leads the movement and how should it lead? Obviously the head leads, but what is the sequence after that? Some people might say the hip, others the knee, and both are good guesses. In fact it is the knee, but first the ankle needs to be released. It's very hard to let the ankle bend if it's stiff or held; release it and then release the back of the knee. The resulting bend allows the thigh to swing forwards freely in a pendulum-like motion from the hip.

The next time you go out for a walk and have to stop for some reason, see how smoothly you can take that first step as you set off again. Keep breathing, and try to iron out the bumps as you begin to move. By learning to become a 'conscious walker', you are now well on your way to becoming a 'conscious runner'.

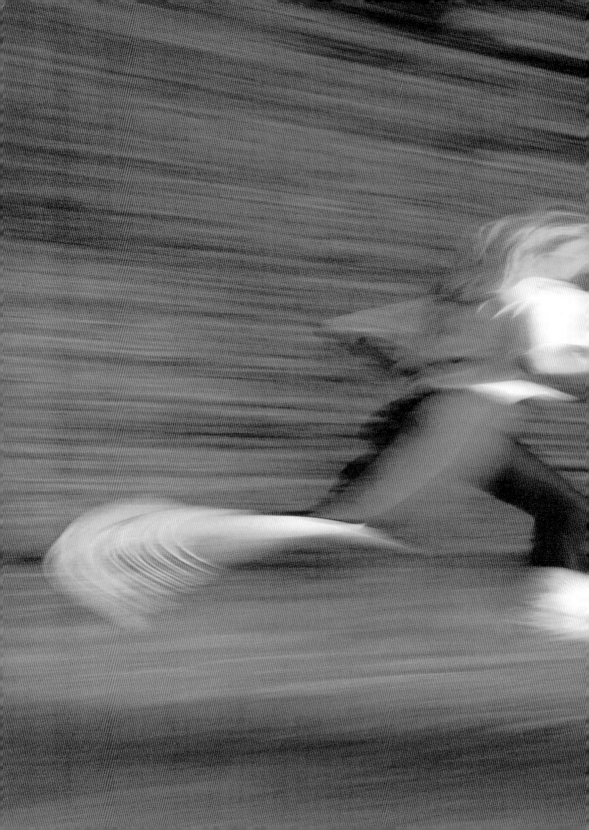

4

BUILDING THE FOUNDATIONS

'Running is not an affair of applied mechanics or economic necessity but an expression by the human body of rhythm and grace and strength which, at its best, rises above the immediate and practical requirements of a given race.'

W. R. Loader, **Testament of a Runner**

Let's work our way through the parts of the body involved in the act of running.

Put simply, running consists of placing one leg in front of the other. As we saw earlier, this simple act can be performed in many different ways, some better than others. To help us understand what distinguishes 'good' running, we need to study the concepts of independence and dynamic stability.

Independence is the ability to move one bit of the body without having to move everything else. (Anyone who has ever had a crick in their neck, which necessitated turning their whole body in order to see over their shoulder, knows the value of this.) A coordinated activity such as running requires independence of the legs from the torso, the arms from the torso, the head from the neck and the eyes from the head.

The typical pattern of many runners involves 'posturing oneself' by tightening the torso so that it is held in place with a lot of muscular tension. The advice commonly given in running magazines and books, and by many doctors and physiotherapists, is to develop the abdominal and back muscles to 'support' the torso. Sometimes corrective measures are recommended, such as tilting the pelvis or tucking in the chin.

The problem with this approach is that it tends to pull things towards each other – as in the case of the sit-up, where the ribs are pulled towards the pelvis; the pelvic tilt, which pushes the pelvis into the legs; and the chin tuck, which pulls the head into the neck. A tendency to tighten or fix has at least three negative effects: it makes it harder to breathe, it makes it

harder to move, and it makes us less aware of what is going on in our bodies.

Runners often have a tendency to 'collapse' – not just after finishing a tough race or workout, but during the act of running itself. It's debatable whether this is based on the idea that running is an activity for the legs so we can let the rest of the body take a breather, or a faulty concept of 'running relaxed', or a lack of awareness regarding the interrelation of the legs and torso. Whatever the reason, the result is the same: independence and potential are reduced, and more effort and energy are required.

The best option is to create stability in the torso – the head-neck-back relationship that we have already explored is ideally dynamic in nature, with the head remaining poised on top of the spine and the back tending to lengthen and widen. The result is a state of 'dynamic stability', characterized by expansion rather than contraction.

The combination of good use and good mechanics results in what we might call 'natural running'. This doesn't mean wearing cotton underwear or flinging your arms about like some flower child from the 1960s, but finding a way to collaborate with or even exploit the laws of nature to your advantage. More specifically, it implies a constructive response to the most

Right Form analysis: **1** foot landing underneath torso; **2** landing leg is slightly bent to cushion impact; **3** swing leg pulled underneath hip, back lengthening – running tall; **4** head poised on top of spine; **5** eyes looking out (not down); **6** arms bent at 90 degrees, wrists toned, arm swing not crossing the midline.

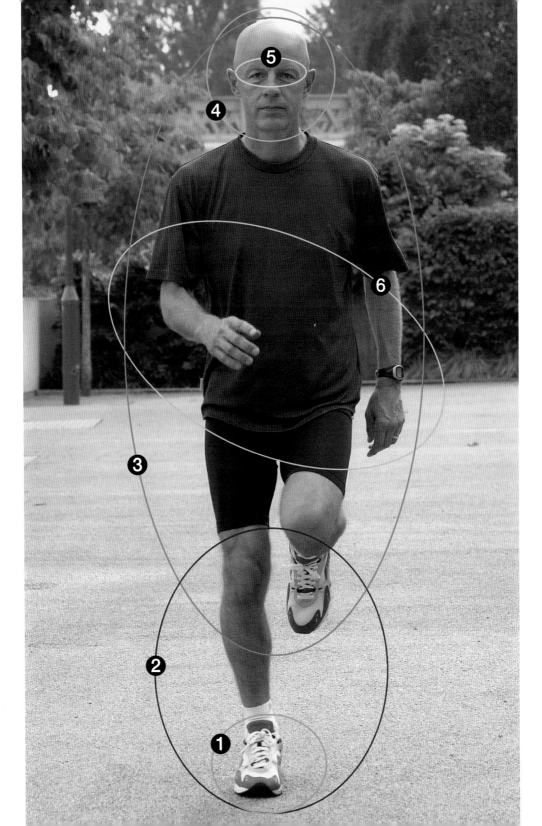

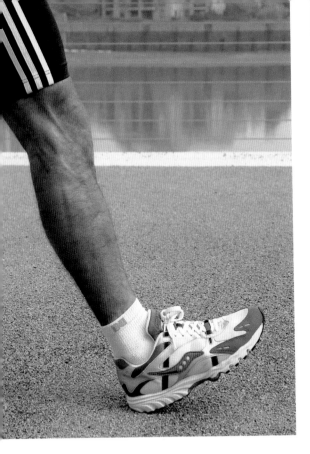

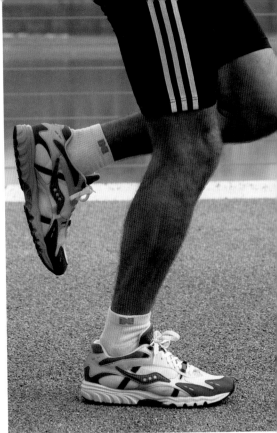

Above Landing on the heel with a straight leg in front of the body, promoted as 'natural' and efficient, actually increases braking forces.

Above Landing on the front of the foot, with the foot directly underneath the body, reduces braking forces and improves efficiency.

powerful force in the universe – no, not compound interest, but the force of gravity. The challenge for the 'natural runner' is to find a way to let gravity assist in initiating and maintaining forward momentum, and to reduce, as much as possible, what exercise physiologists term 'braking forces'.

1. Feet first

So how do you learn to run with the brakes off? First, this raises the thorny question of where and how your foot lands as you run. Think back to our models of running in Chapter 1. If conventional running wisdom is to be believed, we are meant to land on the heel of the foot. This view is backed by shoe manufacturers who do us the favour of equipping most running footwear with thick air- or gel-padded heels to help cushion the shock of landing – a force that can be five-times body weight, or even more if you really like to stomp.

The problem with landing on the heel is that the foot first touches the ground in front of the body. This is what causes the braking action, as anyone who has tried to slow a descent down a steep slope by digging their heels in will attest. Unfortunately, braking forces not only slow our forward progress, making us work harder to maintain pace, they also increase stress and shock to the system. This can hardly be called 'natural running'. According to Clyde Hart, coach to the great Michael Johnson: 'Foot placement is the key to speed. Many athletes place a foot slightly in front of their centre of gravity and that actually causes a blocking effect. It's like they're putting the brakes on all the time.'

It is nearly impossible to land under the centre of gravity if you put your heel down first. Instead of landing on the heel, consider the idea of letting the forefoot touch first. This doesn't mean landing on your toes like a ballerina. In fact, the whole foot can easily touch the ground on landing as long as your weight is on the forefoot. There's a simple test for this: stand with your weight well on your heels and try to lift them off the ground. Impossible. Now shift your weight forward on to the balls of your feet by tilting slightly from your ankles. From this position, it should be relatively easy to raise your heels off the ground – this shows you where you need to land.

Warning: it is possible for the forefoot to touch down first but still land too far in front. There are a couple of runners who live near me, with the biggest calves you've ever seen, who are guilty of this!

Another way to improve your ability to distinguish your heel from your forefoot is to practise bouncing. Besides being a useful component of a warm-up, this is a great way to develop quickness and elastic recoil. With knees slightly flexed and the weight on the balls of your feet, do your imitation of the Ali Shuffle. Now compare that with a bit of Rope-A-Dope, where the weight is on your heels. As you bounce on the balls of your feet, you can try different patterns: forwards, backwards, sideways, both feet on the ground, then just one. You can also take this into movement for 5–10 m (16–32 ft) or so.

Learning to skip like a boxer helps to develop the ability to bounce on the forefoot. There are all kinds of patterns and variations you can try to make this as fun and challenging as you please. The key is to help the nervous system develop speed of response, so that you know how to get your feet off the ground as quickly as possible. Good runners spend as little time on the ground as they can and are therefore able to take advantage not only of gravity, but also of the energy return from each landing. If you leave your foot on the ground too long, that free boost will go.

2. Timing

Get your timing right and you'll really move. Get it wrong and the additional costs can be huge.

When trying to improve your stride, think about taking quick, light steps; think about running as if you were barefoot on hot sand. This is because the longer you leave your foot on the ground (and we are, it must be said, talking hundredths of a second here), the greater the loss of natural spring in your stride and the more you will start to feel like you are

A runner's experience: Bob

For the first three or four months after attending an Art of Running workshop I worked on the various tasks and tried to apply them to my running, but I finally gave up – I just couldn't get things right.

Strangely enough, it was when I stopped trying to apply what I had learned that I finally 'got it'. I started running the way I had always run, but without thinking I changed and started to run falling forward.

I feel as though I am running much more efficiently and I haven't had a single injury since. It has also made running much more fun. I feel as though I am improving, while before it was just a downward path to sixty-plus.

driving on flat tyres. In addition, you will have to wait longer for gravity to give you a free pull. It's like adding another couple of metres to a hill before you crest it and get pulled down the other side.

Runners who wait too long to get their feet off the ground are often trying to feel their foot land before giving the command to remove it. By the time the message gets through to the foot, the crucial moment has passed and they are too late. On the other hand, runners with more practice and experience can give themselves a direction before the act itself. This means thinking about getting your foot off the ground before it actually touches down. You actually feel the aftermath of what has just occurred. This is useful for adjusting future strides but is not particularly helpful in guiding the immediate step.

For an analogy, start tapping your finger on the table in a quick rhythm. The mere thought is enough to launch the action and the sensation of your finger pressing against the wood will tell you that things are going as planned. Now tap again – but wait until you feel the finger touch the table before reacting. Too slow, right? If you watch a group of mixed-ability runners, you will notice a whole range of reaction times. Some runners seem to touch lightly and rapidly, as if they are gliding over the ground like bugs skating across a pond. Others appear heavy

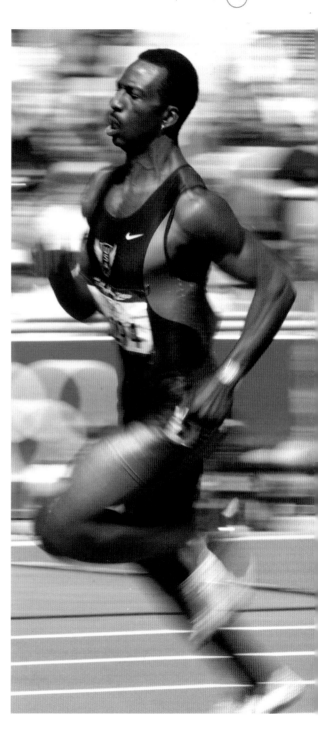

MICHAEL JOHNSON ▶
World record holder at 200 m and 400 m but with a style criticized as 'unnatural' during his era, Johnson is now viewed as the epitome of running efficiency.

and rooted to the ground. The first are skimmers, the second are plodders.

If you want to work your way up the running food chain, this is one area where you will need to practise and improve. Here are some of the qualities that will make progress probable, and hopefully more enjoyable:

- A good idea of what's required: clarity of intention;
- Acceptance of the fact that what you think you are doing may be quite different from what is really happening;
- Patience, perseverance and a sense of humour to see you through the steep part of the learning curve.

In return, you will develop greater elastic strength and increase your speed of reaction, creating a nervous system that gets the message to the right places post-haste.

3. Running tall

Most, though by no means all, running coaches extol the value and importance of 'running tall' in order to achieve optimal performance. One such, Tim Galloway, identifies ten benefits of running with good posture. These include running more easily, suffering fewer injuries, and breathing more efficiently. Coaches try different means to encourage runners into this state, and Galloway cites the advice of the great New Zealand coach Arthur Lydiard. He suggested that we should imagine a pulley attached to our breastbone, with a rope running through it to the top of a small building a block away; the

rope is pulling us towards the top of the building as a way of helping us to lift the chest as we run. He also suggested that we should imagine ourselves suspended from a thread attached to our heads, like puppets. (I once had a coach try and pull me up by my hair, but neither coach nor hair are still with us…)

In Western society, however, it is sad but true that it is much more the norm to slump than to possess the beautifully lengthened back of the tribesman. Indeed, it is extremely rare to find someone who, when asked to stand at full height, does not immediately assume some variation on a military stance: the neck is tightened and the head pulled into the spine, causing it to compress, while the chest is raised, causing the lower back to tighten and hollow and the knees and legs to stiffen. This 'posture' requires considerable effort to maintain. Runners are by nature a persistent lot and many, to their detriment, will try to incorporate some variation of this into their running. The result is a far cry from the natural, efficient poise we are seeking.

4. Head

We've established the idea that the head leads and the body follows. Now consider that the head weighs at least 4.5 kg (10 lb), depending on how great a runner you think you are. The relationship of the head to the torso is therefore of vital importance. If we think back to

Right The ability to maintain the integrity of the head-neck-back pattern is challenged (and strengthened) by learning to lean 'up' while you lean forward.

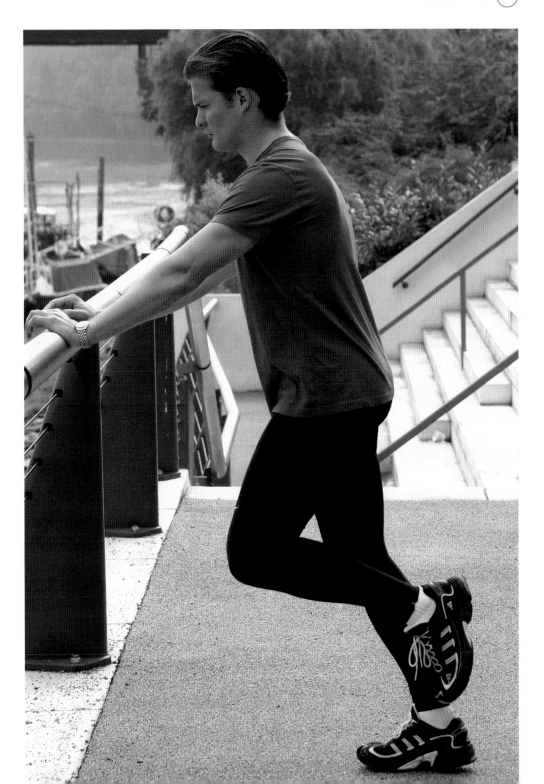

Alexander's discoveries, we know that disturbing the natural balance of the head, either by pulling it back and down or thrusting it forwards, will have a major impact on performance. Unfortunately, film directors don't understand this. Watching *Chariots of Fire* again recently, I was amazed by Ben Cross's depiction of Harold Abrahams at the 1924 Olympics: head thrown back and eyes closed in ecstatic anticipation of winning the 100 m gold medal. Fat chance outside the cinema! (In fact, photographs of the race suggest that Abrahams maintained good technique right to the finish line.) Practise this at your peril...

No wonder the Kenyans are such great runners – look at their mothers! Kenyan women can carry remarkably heavy loads on their heads with no loss of poise, and walk for considerable distances over varied terrain without losing their equilibrium. This highlights the important role that the balance of the head plays in movement.

5. Eyes

The head, as we've just seen, is a heavy object. Runners generally like to look down. The connection is obvious.

When asked why they focus on the tarmac, most runners say it's to avoid stepping in dog

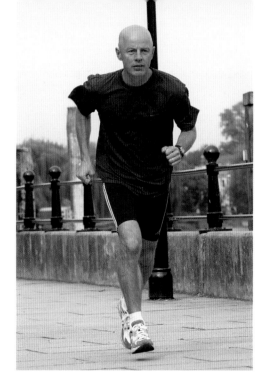

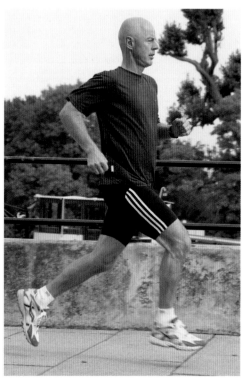

Above right Pushing or dropping the head forward brings a downward pressure, creating shortening along the front of the torso. This restricts breathing and puts strain on the lower back.

Right When we run, while the external direction is horizontal, the internal direction (line of force along the spine) is vertical. Ideally, the head leads and the body follows.

mess or to make sure they don't trip on an uneven surface. Both reasons have some validity, but in practice runners look down as the rule and look ahead as the exception. If you ask someone to keep their head still while looking first to the right and then to the left, there is a tendency for their head to follow the movement of their eyes. And when it comes to looking down, most people like to tilt the head from the base of the neck. So what effect does looking down have on the runner?

● Running heavily

Runners who look down tend to run more heavily. When I ask runners to rate the impact of their foot on the ground on a scale from 1–10 (light to heavy), first when looking down and then when gazing into the distance, they invariably rate the impact as lighter when they are looking ahead.

'Running heavy' is associated with various foot, shin and leg problems; also with the oft-heard warning: 'Running jars your spine.' I remember one runner I worked with who could be heard hitting the ground enthusiastically as he went along. When asked if he was aware how hard he landed, he said that he was – but that it was much better than before. When asked to elaborate, he recounted how, two-thirds of the way

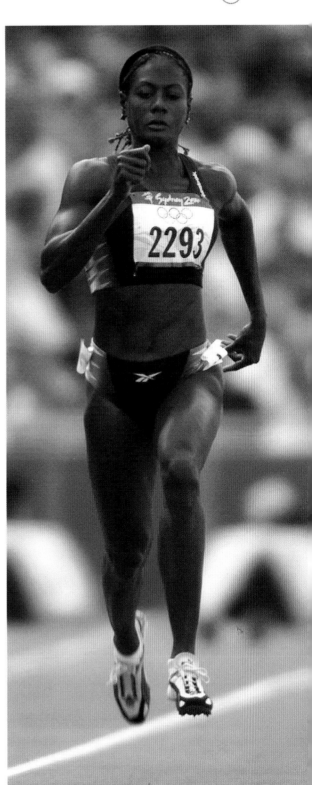

MERLENE OTTEY ▶

The great Jamaican sprinter demonstrating independence between her eye direction – looking down – and her head, which is going up. For most runners, where the eyes go, the head follows.

through a 30-km (18½-mile) race, he started to feel the pain of his efforts. So in a bid to maintain his pace, he consciously started to drive his feet into the ground – as he put it, to 'pound through the pain'. The result was that he pounded his way into a stress fracture, which kept him sidelined for six months.

● **Neck and shoulder pain**

As an experiment, try holding a 4.5-kg (10-lb) weight out in front of you for a while. It takes a lot of effort. When the head is tilted forwards from the base of the neck, it puts tremendous strain on the neck and shoulders – which have to work very hard to keep the head from falling off and hitting the ground. This problem is compounded when the runner, in an effort to see ahead, looks up by pulling the head back and increasing the curve and strain on the neck and spine. This tendency can lead to the development of a hump at the base of the neck.

● **Shortening the body**

Looking down encourages runners to lean forwards and to shorten the front of their bodies. Research has shown that runners who lean too far forward tend to cut an inch off their stride – which will add minutes to their marathon time. Runners who lean forward and shorten the front of the body also tend to have more difficulty breathing, something most would surely like to minimize!

In contrast, looking ahead gives the brain sufficient time to see what's coming up, and tell the feet what to avoid and how to adjust. This is particularly important for runners who train on uneven surfaces – or who just wish to avoid the dog mess.

Improvement, however, may not be what you perceive it to be. I worked with a runner who realized that he had always looked down when he ran. He then made a 'simple' change and, heeding my advice, kept his eyes focused 30–50 m (98–164 ft) down the road. However he didn't recognize that when he looked down, he tended to drop his head along with his neck. His 'improvement' involved pulling his head back but leaving his neck where it was. This meant that he now ran with his face forward but was still hunched over, and his neck was completely scrunched in the process.

6. Arms

It's amazing how many runners plod along with their arms held stiffly and stuck to their sides. What little movement there is often involves the shoulders, so that the whole torso rotates with every stride. Running in this way is like driving with the handbrake on: you are always working against yourself.

Contrast this with the arm movement exhibited by many top runners: elbows bent at 90 degrees, wrists neither floppy nor rigid, and arms moving backwards and forwards, sometimes coming slightly across the body but with very little rotation in the torso. When the arms are used in a coordinated and rhythmic fashion, they are a wonderful source of power and energy. How much does a runner lose by not taking advantage of them?

Try this simple experiment to get a sense of how much you may be robbing yourself. First, find a gentle hill 30–50 m (98–164 ft) long. Hook your thumbs in your waistband and run up the hill. Notice how much energy this takes and how hard the legs have to work. Return to the bottom of the hill and run up it, but this time energize your arm swing. Which was easier? If you are like most runners, the latter experience will be much more to your liking.

Freeing the arms and legs

The shoulder and hip joints are designed to allow the arms and legs, respectively, to function independently of the torso. This means, for example, that we can lift or swing our arms without having to move the torso. One of the qualities seen in great runners is that the head and torso stay quiet (yet dynamic) while the arms and legs do their thing.

An interesting test of independence can be performed in a supine position, with the knees bent. Lift an arm over your head and note whether or not this movement causes any major changes in the neck or back, such as tightening or twisting. Repeat with the other arm, and then try the same procedure with the legs. Gently lift your right foot off the floor and then extend the leg so that it ends up stretched out. Most people find that the back tends to compensate when they try this. In fact, it should be possible to lift the leg and stretch it without any tightening of the abdomen or rolling of the pelvis.

The benefit of this procedure is that you will become aware of the lack of independence

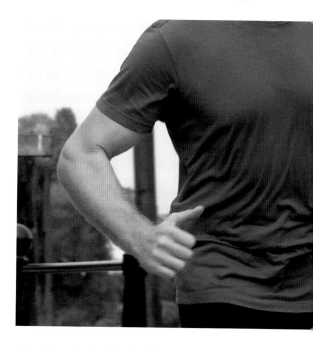

Above Excess tension in the thumbs – here held rigidly by the runner – can further manifest itself by tension in the shoulders.

between the limbs and the torso, a lack which will be hidden during movement. By learning to reduce it, you should be able to run more freely.

Torso

Many great runners allow their shoulders to rotate slightly around the spine with each swing of the arm. This reflects the body's ability to rotate in a 'double spiral' pattern around the spine, providing the body is not held stiffly in place. A child reaching for a toy will demonstrate this; you may also notice it when shaking hands.

This rotation is balanced by a counter-rotation in the hips, so that when the left knee goes forwards (hips thus spiralling to the right) it is balanced by the right arm (upper torso spiralling to the left). This spiral action is what connects the movement of the arms to the movement of the legs in running. Some of the ways we prevent this natural movement are by 'postural fixations' such as carrying things in the arms, or 'pulling down' when we sit slumped at a computer.

The spiralling action is facilitated by the atlanto-occipital joint in the neck, which enables us to turn our head freely without having to move the shoulders. It also allows us to rotate the shoulders and torso while the head remains still and poised. Without this joint, every time the body turned, the head would be obliged to follow, like someone with a crick in their neck, or an amateur shoplifter.

Crucially, this spiralling action works best when the spine is at an optimal length. In other words, when we really are 'running tall'.

Breathing

Early in his career, Alexander was known as the 'Breathing Man', because he was able to help people improve in this area. He concluded that you could not improve a person's breathing without improving their use. 'I learned from these experiences,' he wrote, 'that I could not enable my pupils to control the functioning of their organs, systems or reflexes directly, but that by teaching them to employ consciously the primary control of their use I could put them in command of the means whereby their functioning generally can be indirectly controlled.'

In running magazines and books, you often read that runners should 'belly breathe'. The reasons for this are (a) to counteract the bad habit of pulling the belly in when inhaling (thereby interfering with the natural movement of the diaphragm) and (b) to use more lung capacity than one would by simply breathing with the chest. Taken at face value, this seems like reasonable advice, which should be simple enough to carry out.

However, my personal experience highlights the dangers of trying to improve your breathing in this way. After reading about the benefits of belly breathing back in the 1970s, I dutifully put it into practice during preparation for various marathons. Along the way, I also developed a chronic ache in my lower back. Eventually I made the connection between the way I was belly breathing and the pain I was suffering. I realized that in pushing my abdomen out with every inhalation (twenty or so times per minute), I was arching my lower back and creating strain in that area.

This was exacerbated by the fact that I was clinging to another piece of common advice: that you must strengthen (in other words, tighten) the abdominal muscles to avoid back problems. So there I was, trying to push my belly out against those tight abs – a ludicrous notion, but not unusual in the world of the quick fix. To see what I mean, try pushing out your belly when you inhale and see if you feel your lower back tighten or arch. Now, tighten your stomach and try to push it out when inhaling. Do you notice anything else getting involved, like your neck and shoulders?

Since the bottom of the lungs is about 7 cm (3 in) below the nipple, there isn't any way of getting air into the abdomen short of being shot! So the very term 'belly breathing' is open to misinterpretation. When the diaphragm (the muscle that does most of the work) descends during an in-breath, it pushes down on the organs of the abdominal cavity, causing the cavity to expand. The whole torso, including the back, expands during the in-breath, not just the abdomen. If you try to push the abdomen out, you may well be preventing the rest of your torso from participating in the movement of breathing in the way that it was designed to do.

Instead of pushing the belly out to prevent it tightening during inhalation, you need to learn to release it during this phase of breathing. In my experience, it is really hard to tighten your abdomen (to support the back) and release at the same time (in order to breathe)! However, if you learn to lengthen your torso as you run, your abdomen will naturally respond to the rhythm of your breathing as well as providing whatever other support is required. In fact, as previously mentioned, it isn't just your abdomen that moves when you breathe, your back also expands in response to the movement of the diaphragm.

What prevents us lengthening the torso? The major culprit is 'pulling down'. When we shorten ourselves, we have to compensate by raising the shoulders, arching the back or lifting the sternum. It is much better to prevent this interference than to add on some new 'improvement'.

In his book, *Mind, Body and Sport*, John Douilliard describes an approach to breathing when running. He suggests that we should learn to breathe through the nose, rather than through the mouth. He points out that breathing through the mouth has several limitations: it is associated with hyperventilation; it tends to be shallower; and it stimulates the sympathetic nervous system, which results in a 'flight or fight' response. This may be useful when avoiding a vicious dog, but is hardly conducive to the sense of release and flow we are seeking on a run. Breathing through the nose, according to Douillard, is what most animals do in their natural state, except under stress (such as when being hunted). It allows air to be filtered; it is generally deeper, meaning more oxygen is made available to our working muscles; and it tends to stimulate the parasympathetic nervous system, which helps to calm us down. There is another interesting effect: breathing through the nose usually helps to lower the heart rate.

When I first tried to breathe through my nose, I found myself constantly panicking and having to gasp in some air through my mouth. I needed to slow down and practise. As I continued the experiments on easy runs, I gradually discovered that my pace was increasing but my heart rate was staying low. As a result, running started to feel less stressful. Eventually, I could run at my 'normal' easy pace and maintain breathing through the nose. This translated into an ability to race with less stress and reduce the cramping I sometimes suffered. Be aware, though, that you can easily put a lot of unnecessary effort

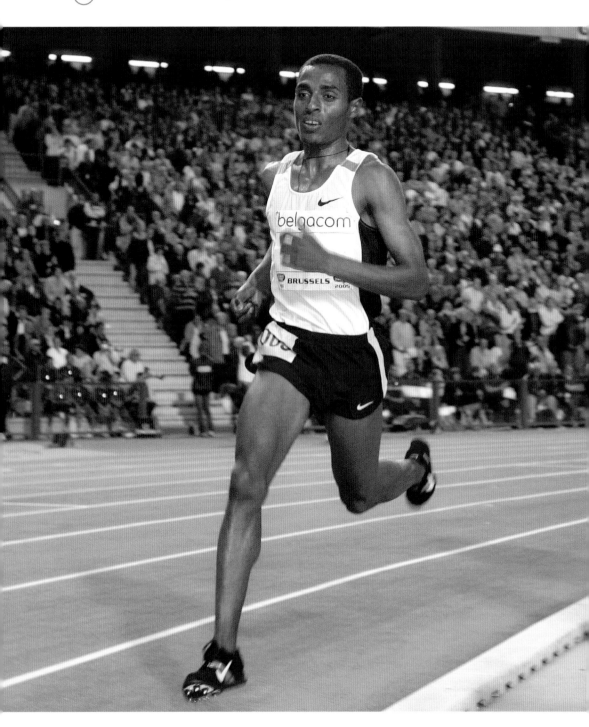

into nasal breathing, which will reduce any benefit you might gain from the practice. Two common habits to avoid are those of sniffing and pulling the head back.

One way to avoid 'end-gaining' during a run, for example running faster than you'd planned, is to pay attention to your breathing rate. For beginners, a general rule of thumb for an easy run is to go at a speed at which you can maintain a conversation. This will help you to stay within your aerobic limits and stop you going into oxygen debt. Jack Daniels, in his book *Daniels' Running Formula*, notes that most elite middle-distance and long-distance runners race at what he calls a 2-2 pace. That is, they either breathe in or breathe out every two steps: right (inhale), left, right (exhale), left, and so on. Slower-paced runs are carried out at a 3-3 or a 4-4 rhythm. Paying attention to your breathing rate can help prevent over-training (which we consider in detail in Chapter 7). As Daniels points out: 'If 3-3 does not provide you with enough air on an easy run, then it's not an easy run. Slow down to where 3-3 is comfortable.'

Finally, it is important to remember that it is impossible to improve your breathing without improving your use. If you allow your ribs to move as nature intended, you will breathe properly. You have to learn to let them move, and you must not hold the ribs and torso in a rigid position.

◀ **KENENISA BEKELE**
The Ethiopian Olympic 10,000 m champion and three times winner of both short and long events at the World Cross-Country Championships demonstrates the easy efficiency that has allowed him to rival even the great Haile Gebrselassie.

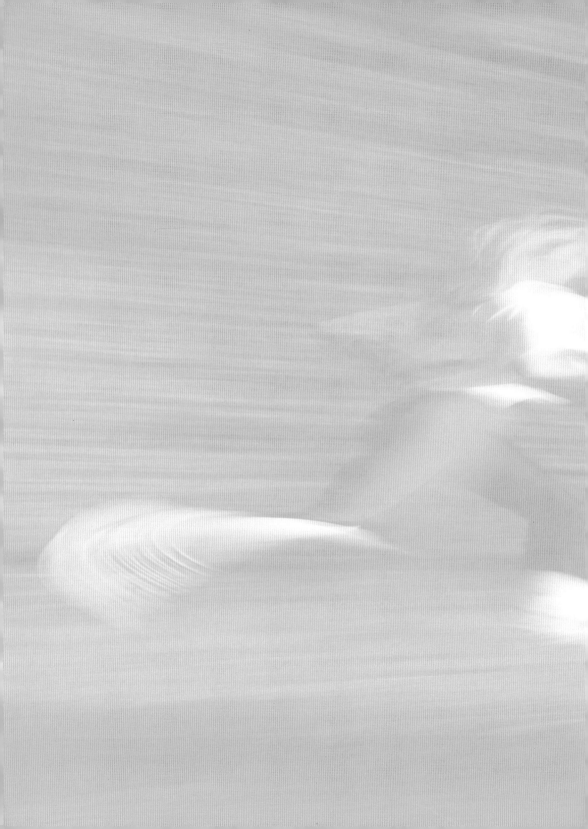

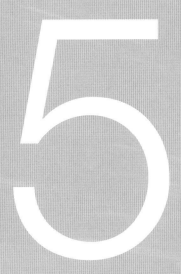

THINKING INTO TRAINING

'Any workout which does not involve a certain minimum of danger or responsibility does not improve the body – it just wears it out.' **Norman Mailer**

When the tone in the neck allows the head to be poised on top of the spine in such a way that the spine is encouraged to lengthen, we function better and move more freely. We need to keep this definition of 'primary control of use' in mind whenever we train, work out or practise running skills. To help us, we can borrow some of the procedures used in Alexander Technique classes. These help to focus attention on a specific pattern of movement within the context of general coordination while promoting 'good use' – that is, to reduce extraneous movement, misdirected effort and unnecessary tension.

Semi-supine

It may seem strange to consider training by lying down calmly rather than by getting up and moving, but ten minutes spent in a semi-supine position can greatly benefit runners. Lie on a firm surface (a mattress or sofa are too soft) in a quiet space with your legs bent, knees pointing towards the ceiling. Rest your hands alongside your lower abdomen, with the elbows pointing out to the side. Support the back of your head with a couple of paperback books, to a comfortable height of about 5 cm (2 in). Keep your eyes open. Here are ten great reasons for lying down once or twice a day:

- **To release unnecessary tension**
  It's also an opportunity for a break from the stresses and pressures of everyday living.

- **To reconnect with your body**
  Except for the daily demands of the stomach, bladder and lower intestine

(and perhaps the odd nagging injury), runners can remain blissfully unaware of their bodies. In the semi-supine position, you can 'wake up' to what is happening with your body, increasing your ability to respond to feedbackeffectively, both from within (sensations) and without (instructions from a coach).

- **To increase balance and coordination**
  Most of us can improve these. Try this version of the simple test outlined in Chapter 3 to see how 'unbalanced' you are.

  Stand in front of a mirror with your feet fairly close together. Now lift one knee so that you are standing, stork-like, on one leg. How much have you leaned over to one side? If it is more than a degree or two, this indicates a problem. There should be no perceptible shift of weight to the supporting leg. Balance sorts itself out, if we allow it to. We all possess a set of reflexes that will do their job provided that we do not interfere with them.

  One of the most common methods of 'getting in the way' concerns the way we carry our head. If we allow the head to remain poised and free on top of the spine, balance is greatly facilitated. But if we pull the head down, we have to work much harder to achieve the same result. Hence the usefulness of semi-supine work. If it is done properly, it can help to reduce the way we inadvertently interfere with the poise of the head, thereby eliminating one more obstacle in our path to greatness.

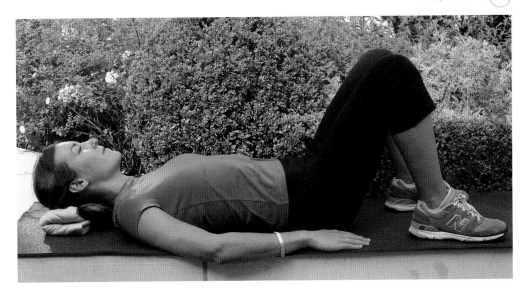

Above The semi-supine position can be practised just about anywhere. With head comfortably supported by a folded towel or a couple of paperback books, this position of 'balanced rest' is a great way to release unnecessary tension and reconnect with your body.

Below Semi-supine can also be used to reawaken our lost sixth sense of kinaesthesia, the ability to sense the position, orientation and movement of our body and its parts. Lying-down work allows us to release strongly contracted muscles and ease us back in touch with ourselves.

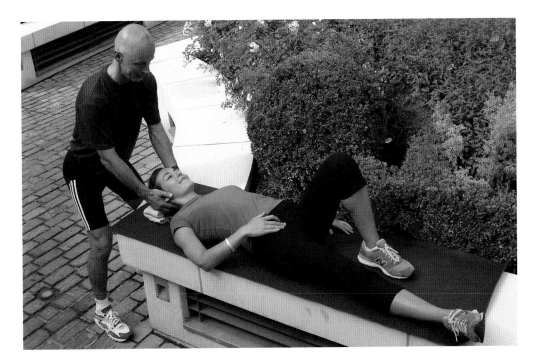

● **To improve breathing**

For many of us, sitting usually involves a degree of collapse. In this state, the ribs end up practically on top of the pelvis, greatly reducing the capacity of the lungs to expand. Breathing then, as a matter of necessity, gets stuck up in the chest. While most of us do tend to reduce our normal slump when we run, our breathing may still be laboured – and it's not because of the pace. It's because the muscles that pull the ribs down have not fully released and have to be worked against. It's a bit like running in a T-shirt that's a couple of sizes too small. Lying down and encouraging the torso to release into lengthening and widening helps to remove this kind of restriction.

● **To give more length**

While running coaches the world over exhort their charges to 'run tall', it's a fact that most of us tend to shorten ourselves. The average person loses around 1 cm (½ in) in height between waking up in the morning and going to sleep at night. This is caused by pressure on the spinal discs and downward pressure in the form of gravity, plus a tendency to pull down or collapse. This literally squeezes the juice out of our spines. The phenomenon can be lessened if we lie down and learn to lengthen ourselves on a regular basis.

● **To improve focus and attention**

Running well, particularly in competition, is related to what sports psychologists call 'arousal' or 'activation level'. If it is too low, we feel sluggish, tired and unmotivated. If it is too high, we feel stressed, pressured and tense. Most of us know when we are 'in the zone' – energized, focused, ready and eager to run well. Lying down can help you become aware of how you are reacting to a forthcoming event (for example, shallow breathing, tension in the neck and shoulders, worries about performing well), while creating the conditions for ideal performance (long spine, relaxed breathing, and a sense of control).

● **To move from rest to activity**

Semi-supine work can help smooth the transition from a sedentary state to a more active one. Rather than forcing the body to respond to our wishes, we can help it prepare gently and thus reduce the chance of injury.

● **To aid recovery**

After a run or training session, we are not always aware of how we have tightened, pulled ourselves down (shortened) or distorted our structure. Lying down after a workout can help to release unnecessary tension and unwanted postural distortion. Left unchecked, these reactions can easily become part of our pattern of use and thus affect other areas of life.

● **To boost energy**

Most of us are not full-time athletes. We can't afford to spend the time between workouts watching DVDs, playing computer games and sleeping. We have to work, go to college, bring up a family, and so on. As a result, our energy may be depleted when it comes to training. Ten minutes, semi-supine, is a non-caffeinated method of rejuvenation.

● To reawaken kinaesthesia

Kinaesthesia is the ability to sense the position, location, orientation and movement of our body and its parts. Tense, over-contracted muscles, fixed joints and long periods of inactivity all tend to reduce this sixth sense, and with it our capacity to 'hear the whispers before they turn into screams'.

According to David Garlick, in his book *The Lost Sixth Sense*, 'As a person becomes aware of his/her muscle state, this lays the basis for better functioning of the musculo-skeletal system and will help to prevent or lessen musculo-skeletal problems. Secondly, there is an important effect psychologically in being aware, even if only every now and again, of one's muscles. There develops a sense of individual unity, of being at peace with oneself, of being "centred" in oneself.' Learning to release strongly contracted muscles through semi-supine work helps undo our tendency to suppress sensory inputs and eases us back in touch with ourselves.

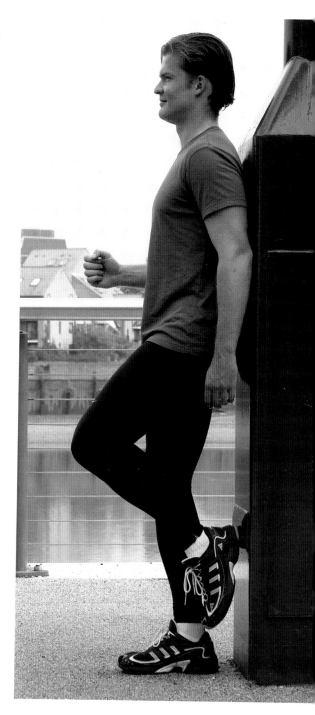

Right Wall-work: the wall provides the runner with feedback on his ability to maintain his length as he balances on one leg while pulling his other foot up underneath him. The next challenge is to repeat this exercise away from the wall, increasing the demands for balance and freedom.

Wall work

Like the floor, a wall can also give great feedback about our use – the way we organize ourselves both at rest and when we move. It can offer an insight into what is happening when we run, and provide the knowledge for making improvements.

Stand with your back to a wall, heels approximately 6 cm (2½ in) away from it. Now let yourself lean back against the wall and see which part of your body touches it first. If it is your head and/or shoulders, it means that you tend to stand (and run) with the pelvis pushed forwards and shoulders tilting back. If your bottom hits first, it means that you tend to stiffen your ankles and legs and reach for the wall with your bottom. Ideally, your shoulders and bottom should arrive at the wall at the same time, and the back of your head should not touch it at all. If your head is touching, it means that you are tightening your neck and pulling your head back. (A runner who loses the ability to cope with the stress of a race will often pull the head back into the neck in a reflex movement known as the 'startle effect'.)

You are now standing with your shoulders and bottom (but not your head) touching the wall. You can use the wall to help orient yourself, and think of your back aiming up the wall and towards the ceiling ('back and up'). This thought can be repeated several times until the experience registers kinaesthetically and you have a sense of what the words mean. This can be helpful to anyone who tends to lean a bit too far forward (and who doesn't?) when they run.

Once you get a sense of 'back and up', add the following:

Give a thought to releasing the front of the ankle and the back of the knee, and roll your right foot up on to the toe. Did anything change as far as your back was concerned? For example, did your hips come away from the wall? If so, this indicates that your hip joint is a little 'stuck', and when your legs moved forwards, they pulled your hips with it. This lack of independence shows up in runners who 'sit on the legs'. The other thing that might have happened is that your right hip collapsed and your body sagged. This lateral displacement of the torso is wasteful and costly. If, however, your knee released forwards and you rolled gently up on your toe while your spine continued to aim back and up, then you're making excellent progress.

Now try alternating one foot with the other and see if you can maintain a sense of dynamic stability in your head and torso. Now try it faster. When this procedure is done well, it encompasses many of the elements found in good running: a long back which tends to stay up and off the legs, a head poised and leading the spine, and ankles and knees that are free – for efficient leg movement, balance, independence and coordination between the top half of the body and the bottom half, with each part working in a synchronized and harmonious manner.

Finally, repeat all this away from the wall! This will increase the demands for balance and freedom, as the wall is no longer there to provide support and feedback.

The lunge

A lunge is like the movement performed by a fencer who is trying to skewer an opponent. The leg in front is bent, while the trailing leg is straight. (This is different from the version taught in many fitness classes, where both knees are bent at 90 degrees and the back knee is aimed directly towards the ground, with the pelvis tucked under.)

When practising the lunge, pay attention to maintaining the relationship between the head, neck and back while letting the front knee bend. Place the emphasis on allowing the head to lead (this is the primary movement), and the leg to bend in response (secondary). This enables the back to lengthen and widen, promoting independence between leg and back.

When you perform this procedure slowly, there is plenty of time to eliminate unnecessary effort and encourage the correct response to take place. So while your head is leading your spine into length, you can ensure that your straight back leg releases and lengthens.

Because the lunge is not that far removed from what we do when we run, this type of stretch can be useful in that we can think the same way 'during the act' and prevent undue shortening in the process. Rather than forcing the front knee to bend any which way, encourage it to release out and away over the toe, again with the same action employed

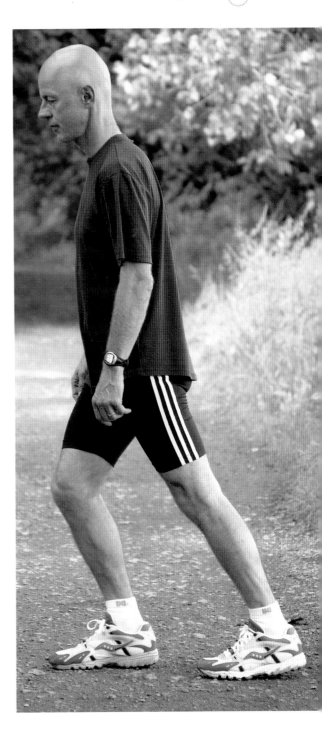

Right The lunge. This looks like the movement performed by a fencer: the front leg is bent while the trail leg is straight. Practising the lunge correctly is a way to discover some of your 'postural eccentricities' and the effect they can have on your running technique.

when running, but with a maximum of freedom and awareness. Indeed, having a clear idea of what we would like to happen when we run is one way of improving our running action. Going out and simply hoping that time and experience will help smooth the rough edges is a slow and often painful journey.

While performing the lunge, you may also discover some postural eccentricities – those little habits your mother adored but which drive coaches to distraction. For example, many of us have no idea how we 'wear our feet': are they pointing straight ahead, at ten to two, or are they at ten to twelve? To develop a good, efficient, injury-resistant stride, it's important to run with the feet pointing straight ahead. 'Toeing-out' not only places unnecessary strain on the rest of the body, it also has implications as far as stride length is concerned. A study showed that runners with size nine feet who toe-out 20 degrees – just 1 cm (½ in) from straight – lose 16 m (52 ft) during the course of a 1-km (0.62-mile) run. If you extend this over a marathon, it adds up to more than 400 m (1,312 ft) – which could make a considerable difference if you were close to breaking the three-hour barrier.

SEBASTIAN COE ▶

Sebastian Coe demonstrating control, balance and power on a tough hill climb. The increase in difficulty caused by running uphill is a good way to challenge your coordination and the integrity of your head-neck-back relationship. The skill is to prevent it becoming a test of strength and endurance by maintaining length through the spine and avoiding tightening the neck.

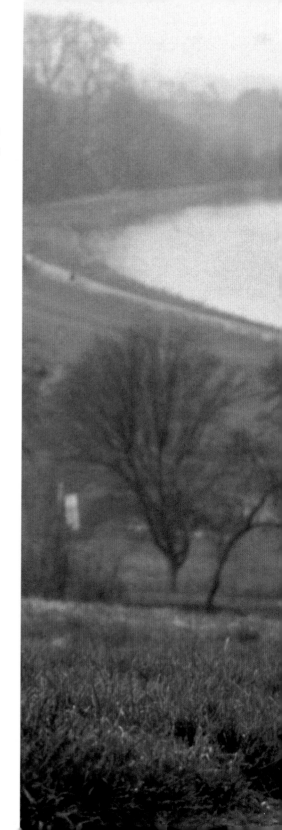

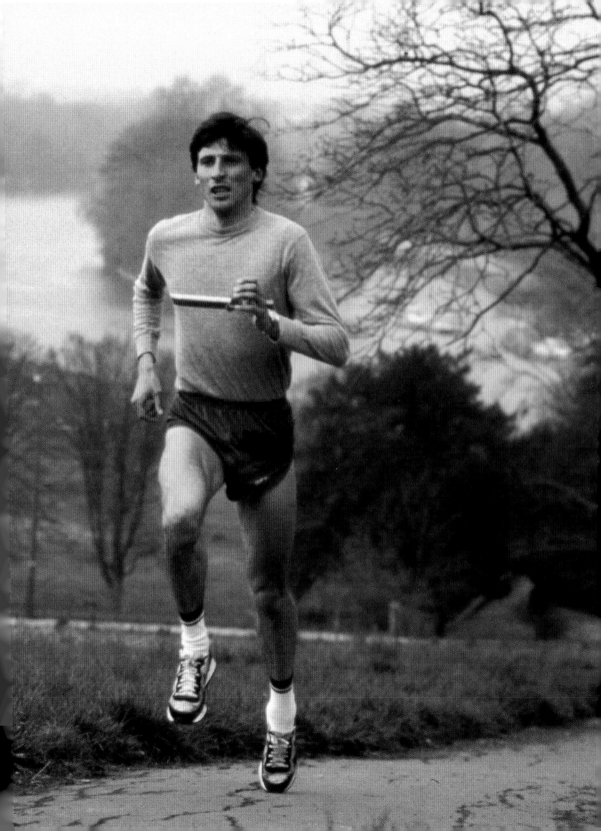

Drills

Drills are an important part of training sessions for most club athletes. Ideally, they should be used by every runner. They're like scales and arpeggios in music: they help you warm up, develop a kinaesthetic picture of the correct stride pattern, and improve your running technique.

However, just as scales and arpeggios can become a tedious grind when you've played them a thousand times before, so drills can work against a runner by reinforcing existing patterns of poor coordination and misuse. It's important to approach them with the same attention and intelligence you are now applying to other aspects of your running.

● **Stimulus**

Drills work as a stimulus for greater coordination. Most drills make it harder to maintain a state of general coordination. For example, it is more difficult to run lifting your knees in front of you than to walk. However, this increase in difficulty can inspire you to greater heights of coordination: learning to do hard things well can help you do easy things better. You can also use drills to challenge your powers of coordination. We have already met the lunge, but in order to strengthen your head-neck-back relationship, try running slowly up a hill for 10 m (33 ft), moving your arms and legs in a kind of march. The aim is to maintain length through your spine, and not to tighten the neck or allow the head to pull back. However, trying to go uphill in such a fashion

may cause you to suddenly forget your back and start to focus on your legs. The whole experience then becomes much more difficult on every level, and may quickly degenerate into a test of strength and endurance. This should be avoided. When you focus on your back and continue to lengthen it, the result is one of effortlessness and flow. I have seen many non-runners perform this procedure and be absolutely astonished to find themselves at the top of a 40-m (131-ft) hill with none of the expected fatigue – in fact, they are not even out of breath! It is as though the back, rather than the legs, has taken them upwards. As one said, 'It was like I found my internal spring.'

● **Provocation**

Drills can serve as provocation. For example, I might tell a runner that he is looking a bit slow and weak today – just before I ask him to run a 100 m (328 ft) acceleration. If the runner I am trying to 'provoke' takes the bait and tries to show me what he can really do, he is liable to forget everything he knows about form and just hammer it. After he finishes, I will take the opportunity to point out that he put far more effort and unnecessary movement into that sprint than was really needed. New information such as this can be very useful in assisting a runner's efforts to improve his form, by helping him become aware of what he really does, as opposed to what he thinks he does. If, on the other hand, he inhibits his instinctive reaction and maintains good form while

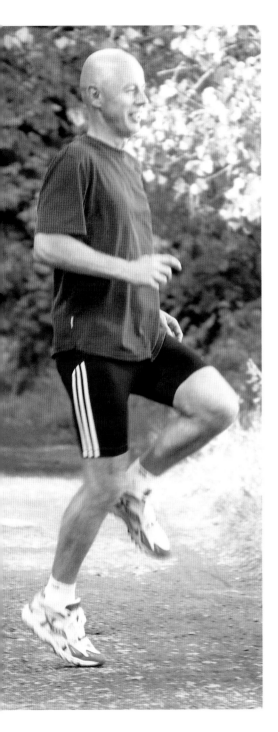

increasing speed in an intelligent manner, this will serve him well when, for example, the need to accelerate presents itself in a race. Frank Shorter wrote of the great Finnish runner, Lasse Viren, 'He had a very smooth stride that essentially did not change as he accelerated in the final laps. Unlike most distance runners, he did not switch to a sprinter's gait in a furious drive to the finish. Somehow he was able to maintain his form and simply run faster. It was all rpm – his leg rate quickened, which made his speed deceptive.' Viren is the only athlete to win the 5,000 m and 10,000 m at two Olympic Games, achieved in 1972 and 1976.

● Integration

Drills can integrate good form – that is, good use – with good running mechanics. Some drills are designed to highlight a certain phase in the stride cycle. For example, bottom kicks (see page 98) are part of the forward swing phase in the cycle and high knees (see page 96) are part of the recovery or float period. Drills such as these can help runners to develop a correct stride pattern. Problems arise when the emphasis is placed on leg movement at the expense of the head-neck-back pattern. This is putting the cart before the horse – otherwise known as that terrible monster, 'end-gaining'.

Left High knees: softening behind the knees while pulling your ankle up underneath the hip brings a dance-like quality to this drill. The particular challenges are to lift the thigh parallel to the ground without 'losing the height' and to avoid leaning back.

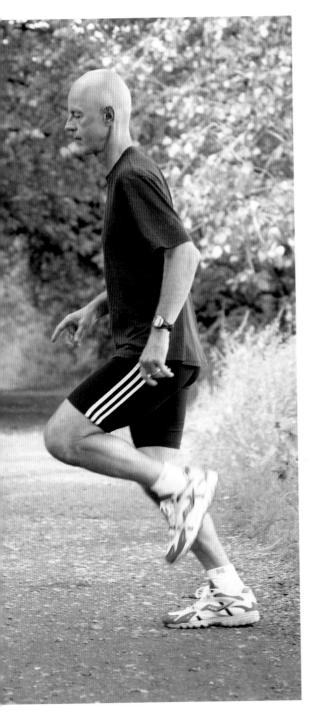

Drills are a stimulus that you must learn to inhibit and direct. For example, when you do the high knees drill, think about not leaning backwards in the process. Try lifting a knee parallel to the ground – you will notice an urge to lean back. However, this is not necessary – the leg can move independently from the torso. So, rather than forcing the knee to come up to waist height, lift it only as far as you can without disturbing the upward lengthening (verticality) of the torso. As your skill and flexibility increase, you will be able to get the knee up higher.

Here are some drills to practise:

High knees

Ten seconds of running with the knees lifted so that the thighs are parallel to the ground. The challenge is to allow this to occur without 'losing the height'.

High knees at the bottom of a hill

Repeat the above drill for five seconds at the bottom of a hill and then slowly run up the hill in short increments of ten seconds. I like to think of this as a moving lunge. It provides a strong stimulus to maintain a sense of length in the torso. If this occurs, there is little or no sense of effort in the legs – just the opposite of what many runners experience going uphill. When

Left Bottom kicks: practise pulling up the ankle directly underneath your hip in order to kick the underside of your bottom with alternate heels. This drill is not an excuse to arch the lower back and pull yourself down! Go slowly and avoid forcing the movement.

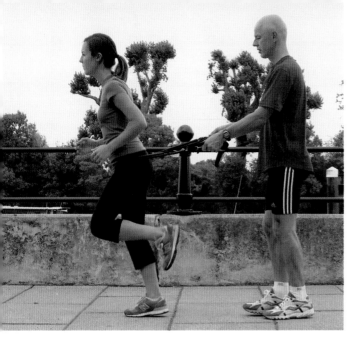

Left To develop the sense of falling and using gravity to provide forward momentum, a rubber cable supports the runner around her hips allowing her to lean forward and up from her ankle in a safe and controlled manner.

Below The rubber cable provides an added stimulus on the runner's legs as he works against them to lift his foot off the ground while maintaining overall poise.

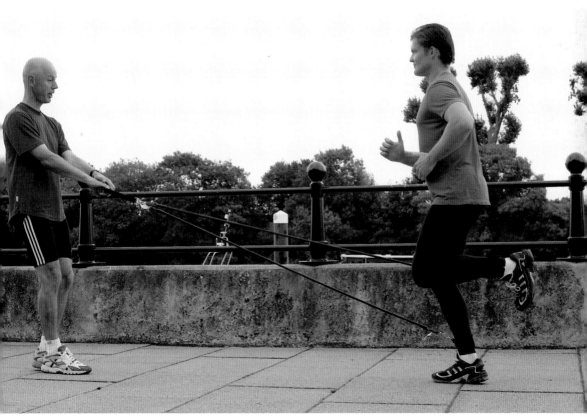

done just before acceleration, it can give a sense of effortless power. The reason for this is that the head and back are leading the movement and the legs are following, not the other way round.

Bottom kicks

Run slowly and allow your heels, alternately, to kick the underside of your bottom. This drill should not be an excuse to arch the lower back and pull yourself down!

Accelerations

Thirty seconds of accelerations, alternated with thirty to ninety seconds of easy running, can be done near the end of a long run. When runners accelerate using their legs, there is a tendency to stiffen the neck, lean backwards and shorten the torso – again, the exact opposite of what is desirable. When runners inhibit this initial impulse but increase the rhythm of their arms, their legs follow suit – with less disturbance to the lengthening of the spine.

Step-overs

This drill helps with the understanding of the concept of circularity in the running stride. It can help you develop a more efficient stride pattern, and reduce wasted time and motion after the foot leaves the ground or toes-off. Lift

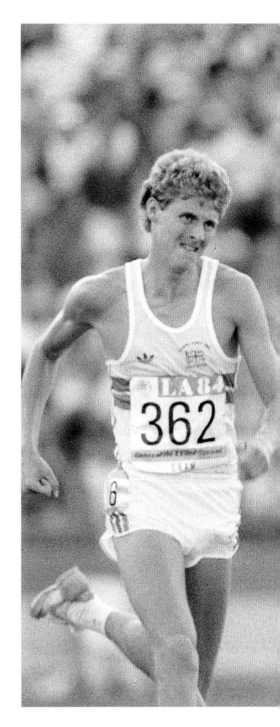

SEBASTIAN COE ▶

The famous battle between Sebastian Coe and Steve Cram in the Los Angeles Olympics 1500 m final. In spite of the visible strain, Coe still manages to maintain his length – and his lead – while Cram's head, neck and shoulders (not to mention the expression on his face) say it all.

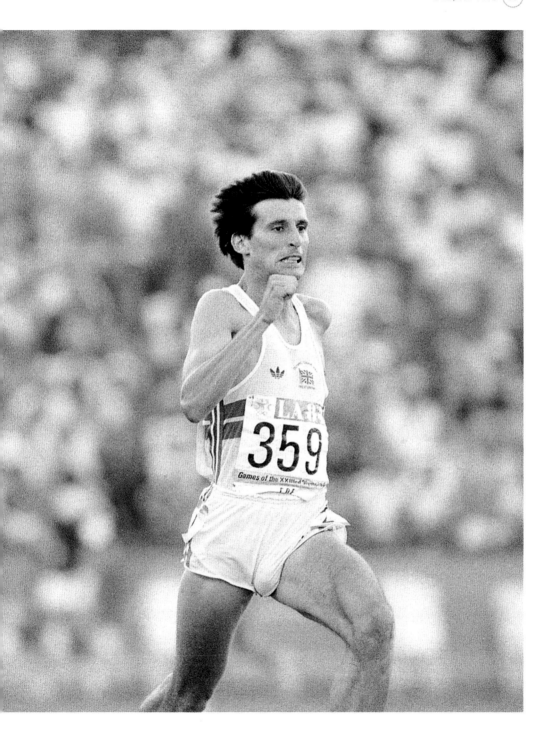

and step with the right foot over the left shin, and place the right foot back on the ground parallel to the left foot (not in front of it). This can be practised while standing still, walking or running slowly, and then at full speed – and, of course, with the opposite leg. The challenge is not to let the technical difficulty interfere with the upthrust along the spine.

Acceleration

Another experiment to try involves what track athletes know as accelerations, usually of 100 m (328 ft). You start slowly and gradually increase the pace, to up to 80–90 per cent of top speed, before easing off over the last 20 m (66 ft). Accelerations are used to warm up and to get used to running at a faster pace.

First, increase speed just by moving your legs faster. Note how much effort this takes. You may also notice that you throw your head back and tighten your shoulders. Now try accelerating a second time by letting your arms lead and your legs follow. This means that each time you move up a gear, you allow the arms to move more quickly in an ever-increasing arc, and your legs follow suit. During this procedure, the head should, of course, remain poised on top of the spine with the shoulders wide open.

If it doesn't work out like that, you are probably trying too hard to get it right. Stop and build up gradually, without worrying about how fast you go at first. You can also reverse the process if you have space, going from fourth gear to first simply by slowing and reducing the movement of the arms without leaning backwards or shortening. Most runners find

this way of 'changing gears' is easier, involves less effort and is much more fun!

Changing pace

We are creatures of habit, and runners have a tendency to always go at the same pace. Once we've reached a certain level of proficiency and fitness, we often chug along on automatic pilot. This can vary from the positively pedestrian to 1.6 km (1 mile) in under 6 mins, depending on our level.

This can be a good thing in that it allows us to think, enjoy the scenery or carry on a conversation without having to attend to the physical and technical requirements of moving. But the trouble with always running at the same pace is that it starts to become mechanical and unconscious. Bad habits become ingrained and disappear into the recesses of awareness. We are no longer in touch with ourselves. In order to continue to enjoy our activity by avoiding injury and boredom, we need to reconnect. We have already seen, in Chapter 2, how our 'end-gaining' tendency causes most of us to run too fast. Here are two examples aimed at the extremes of the running continuum.

For slower runners, it's vital to change gear occasionally. It's not enough to just plod along for thirty minutes, zoning out with your iPod. There are heights of enjoyment you will never experience in that mode. Try picking up the pace – maybe from one tree to the next. Then go back to your normal speed for a couple of trees, and then repeat. Continue like this for five or ten minutes. It isn't a question of exhausting

CASE STUDY
A runner's experience: Neil

By exercising mindfully, my goals have shifted from thrashing out miles and pints of sweat to redirecting the energy somewhere more profitable. The sweat comes as a given! On a treadmill, I've realized how wasteful all that footfall banging and bounding up and down actually is. Exhausting, too.

I've still got upper body issues. I'm a classic case: the more I think about something, the worse it gets! I do things right in drills, but as soon as I get into 'performance mode', the tightness across the clavicle comes back, and my arms stop swinging freely from the shoulder yoke and start coming round in front. My solution is to go back to the basic head-neck-back alignment, think about 'running tall' and allow this to let the shoulders widen and open. It helps, but it needs practice and concentration.

In six months' time, I will be studying my son's first steps thoroughly. I'm sure it will be the first of many occasions when my offspring teach me something!

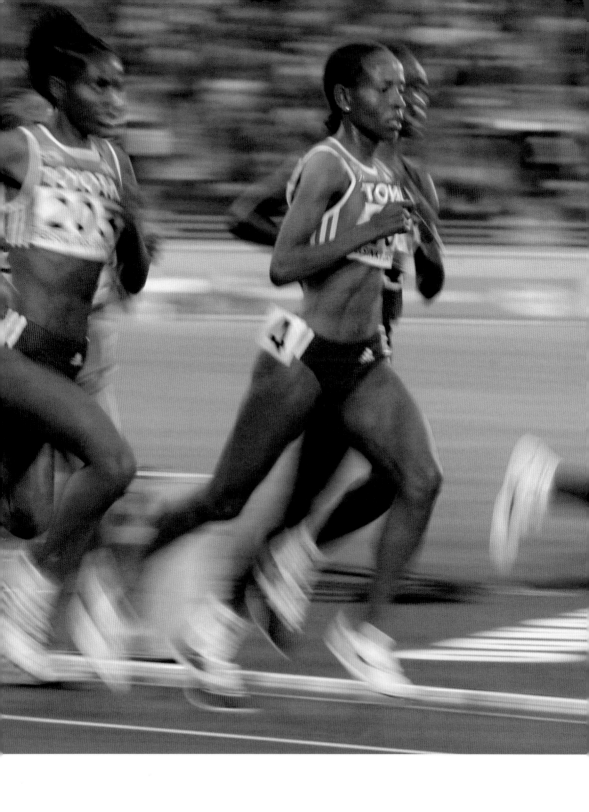

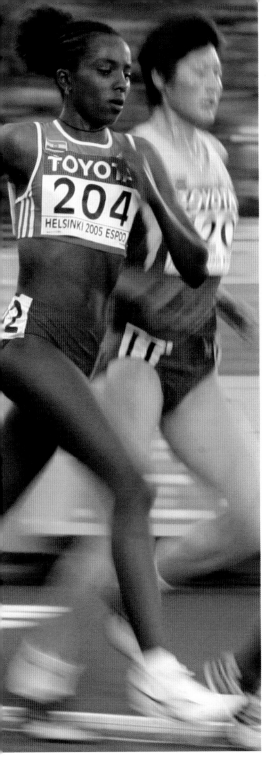

yourself, even though your breathing will quicken and you may initially feel that you are overdoing it; it will cause you to wake up and pay attention to what's going on, getting you to reconnect with the moment and to notice how you are reacting to the stimulus, thereby giving you an opportunity to practise 'thinking in activity'. If at first it seems difficult, unnecessary or even an irritation, it will soon become a source of interest and enjoyment.

For faster runners – those who think going at a pace of anything less than 6 mins 30 secs over 1.6 km (1 mile) is an act of cowardice – try running a couple of minutes slower but with perfect form. Same leg cadence, same movement with the arms and legs, although in a slightly reduced form – in other words, a miniature version of your normal long, flowing stride. The form of many advanced runners deteriorates drastically when they are just out for an easy run or in their warm-up/cool-down phase before or after a race.

A runner I used to nag about paying attention to his stride sent me a note several years later: 'The running stride must be mechanically sound at all times. Often the slow gait of an easy run is entirely inappropriate training for the body. You lean back, run on the

◀ **TIRUNESH DIBABA**

The 2005 world 5,000 m and 10,000 m champion demonstrates poise and grace while competing at the highest level. To race against a field of other elite athletes demands extraordinary attention to what is happening around her, and the ability to react to a change of pace. 'Automatic pilot' is impossible here – and should also be avoided by lesser runners in order to maintain awareness.

heels and use a cadence that programs the mind and body for a slower turnover. You should be using race-cadence in order to condition muscle elasticity and to optimize and harmonize your frequency in preparation for race conditions. This represents a radical change from the way I've always run. I've detected some horrendously inefficient tendencies in my stride: heel striking, no toe drive, dropping the arms, head and shoulders thrown back. And so I have been emphasizing three crucial points during workouts and easy runs: (a) Lead with the upper body, (b) Bounce off the toes, (c) Turnover.'

Video analysis

Any runner who has worked with a coach will know the importance of communication. Whether it's feedback after a training session or a race, the chance to talk through problems or plan ahead, a shoulder to cry on, constructive criticism – all these are vital in a good athlete–coach relationship.

Many coaches use a video camera to assist in training. If you don't work with a coach but still want to see yourself in action, ask a friend to shoot some footage. The images do not lie, and they provide a permanent record of your technique at any given time. You can zoom in for details, and freeze-frame for analysis. You can watch the pictures over and over again. And if you always thought you ran like Haile Gebrselassie, well, maybe this will be proof that you do!

Used skilfully, sensitively and positively, video analysis can be highly motivational for athletes of all standards. However, it also has its pitfalls. It can overemphasize faults, an unnecessary complication for runners whose technique and use may be just fine as they are. Even Olympic champions, studied in super-slow-mo, will show tiny areas needing improvement. However, they have got all day and every day to work on correcting them.

There's also a danger of becoming over-dependent on video, destroying a more instinctive, natural approach to running and making you get bogged down in mechanics. The result, for some, can be 'paralysis by analysis'. Instead of seeing a dynamic, balanced, elegant flowing action, a runner affected in this way will notice only the precise angle of the forearm or a minuscule tilt of a shoulder. Instead of offering scope for improvement through greater self-awareness, the camera merely becomes another factor that nibbles away at self-confidence.

Shoes and running barefoot

A jaundiced definition of running shoes is that of 'coffins for your feet'! In spite of all the advances in shoe technology since the 1970s, the rate of injury among runners has stayed more or less the same. So don't expect a shoe to save you from poor running form, and don't believe everything you read or hear about what a shoe is supposed to do. For example, there is some evidence that anti-pronation shoes actually make the tendency to over-pronate worse! A much better solution is to improve your use, which in turn will help you to prevent your feet from rolling too much.

The difference in the level of feedback gained when running in shoes, compared to running barefoot, is phenomenal. Anyone who has tried the latter will know how much more sensitive one's feet become when unshod. This doesn't mean that everyone should try and imitate the great Ethiopian marathon runner Abebe Bikila and throw their shoes in the bin. But if you can find a safe place to experiment with barefoot running, free of sharp objects and unpleasant animal deposits, have a go.

John Woodward, barefoot runner par excellence, organizes regular Natural Running courses. He exhorts participants to experience the resilience and responsiveness of the foot in its natural state. I found that, even after two hours spent gambolling around the hills, I had no Achilles tendon pain in spite of losing the cushioning under my heel. It also became apparent that runners' strides changed as well, becoming shorter, quicker and less on the heel. Although I do not train barefoot, I have compromised by wearing 'the least amount of shoe' that still enables me to stay injury-free. Training for a marathon in racing shoes left my feet feeling permanently sore, so I went back to a race/trainer model with a little more cushioning. However, whenever possible I take the shoes off and do my warm-up drills or strides barefoot.

Orthotics are another popular and expensive 'solution' to the injury woes suffered by runners. Like some other miracle cures, they can occasionally be life-transforming. However, the results are less spectacular for many other runners in need of help. It's worth remembering the old Zen saying, 'Wherever you go, there you are' – run with bad use and poor technique and you're asking for trouble. In such cases, orthotics may merely help a runner mask more fundamental issues for a while.

Treadmill running

How is running on a treadmill different from running on a non-moving surface – and is it a satisfactory alternative? Personally, I would much rather train outdoors and there is evidence that runners who do so enjoy running more. However, one of the good things about treadmill running in a gym, which can't be replicated in the great outdoors, is that you are often in front of a mirror and can benefit from the feedback it provides. So when the weather is really bad or you don't have access to an outdoor route or indoor track, treadmill running is the next best thing.

The main difference between the two surfaces lies in your relationship with gravity. Because you're on a moving surface, your concern is on not getting pulled off the machine and ending up in a heap! A further complication is that a gym has many distractions from the actual act of running – a bank of screens with personal headphones, perhaps, or a handy holder for your CD player. It's easy, in such a situation, to stop paying attention to your running, which may help to explain the common tendency to run in a more heavy-footed manner and pound the surface.

Nevertheless, you can still get a decent workout – though the possibility of misusing yourself is as much of an issue as it is for outdoor runners. Some treadmill devotees resort to holding on to the handrails to maintain their presence on the device – good for survival, perhaps!

Plyometrics

Plyometrics is a way of helping athletes to develop more power (a combination of strength plus speed) by performing exercises that first make a muscle lengthen (an eccentric contraction), followed as quickly as possible by a contraction (concentric contraction). This is equally relevant whether you're tackling 10 km (6 miles) or 100 m (328 ft). Plyometric training can help strong runners become faster and more flexible by using the strength in their legs more quickly.

The best runners, whatever their distance, minimize the time their feet are in contact with the ground. The longer your feet are down, the more energy you lose from forward movement. One way to measure this is stride rate, or the number of strides you take in a minute. A top athlete will have a stride rate of around 180–210, while a novice's rate will be in the low 160s. In other words, the feet of the elite touch the ground more often, but for less time. Because top athletes are also moving faster, the temptation is to try and emulate them by taking longer strides. However, because we lesser mortals are not as powerful or flexible, we end up over-striding, which is one of the biggest causes of injuries.

Plyometric drills to increase power and flexibility in the legs can help to develop the light, quick running style we're seeking. The basic principle is that by stretching (loading) a muscle before contracting it, the contraction will happen faster and produce a more dynamic effect. To demonstrate this, try a vertical jump from a crouching position. Now do the same thing, but start in a standing position then crouch down before you spring upwards. You should be able to jump higher if you crouch down and then immediately jump up, than if you started from the crouch. This is because your leg muscles have been loaded first.

A classic exercise for improving vertical jumping ability is to step off a bench and, as soon as your feet touch the floor, rebound upwards as quickly as possible. Another method is a press-up with a clap between each repetition. Your pectoral muscles are loaded by the downward force of your body, then the muscles are immediately contracted to push yourself back up.

Running is itself a type of plyometric exercise, in that a runner lands with three to five times his body weight and quickly explodes off the landing foot on to the other foot. Since good runners spend less time on the ground than their inefficient counterparts, it behoves us to develop this aspect of our stride. Remember the idea of running barefoot on hot sand to develop the ability to spend as little time on the ground as possible?

Low-intensity plyometric drills can also be used to awaken the nervous system so that it responds at the ideal rate of 180 strides per minute. After walking for a few minutes, try skipping, hopping on each leg, bounding and tapping your feet on the ground; do not try for height or distance, but for quickness of reaction. After a few minutes of alternating such exercises with walking or easy running, your feet will respond like a tap dancer who has drunk one too many espressos!

Cross-training

Cross-training doesn't mean working out when you're upset. It's the principle of taking part in other sports and fitness activities with the aim of benefiting your primary interest. Here are its plus points:

- **It helps to develop those muscles you don't use when running**

  It gives a well-balanced and toned physique. In particular, strength training – often dismissed as irrelevant by long-distance runners – will increase your lean muscle mass (and won't turn you into the Incredible Hulk). Consequently, cross-training can reduce the risk of injury by taking the stress off muscles that may be tired from running.

- **It aids recovery**

  You can give running muscles a break while still providing a worthwhile training stimulus. This is often referred to as 'active rest'.

- **It adds variety and improves social interaction**

  Running can sometimes be a solitary activity. Joining a group exercise class or playing a weekly game of badminton will give you a new set of sporting friends.

- **It helps runners to improve their use under different circumstances**

  For example, cycling in an aerodynamic position on a road bike can create a great deal of shortening and tension in the neck as you pull the head back in order to see the road. I remember trying to find ways to overcome this problem during my training as an Alexander Technique teacher. Learning how to prevent my head from crunching into my spine as I cycled to my classes paid off years later when a triathlete suffering from tingling and numbness in his hands sought my help. It turned out that an excessive contraction of his neck, perfected during many hours in the saddle, was a major contributor to his problem.

Alexander Technique teachers have, in recent years, begun to explore how the principles of the Technique can be applied to other sports. Perhaps the best example to date is Steven Shaw's brilliant treatise, *The Art of Swimming*, and his development of the Shaw Method of Swimming. The principles of the Alexander Technique are now being applied to activities including rowing, weight training and gym workouts, so there is every opportunity for runners to expand their fitness horizons and reap the benefits of cross-training.

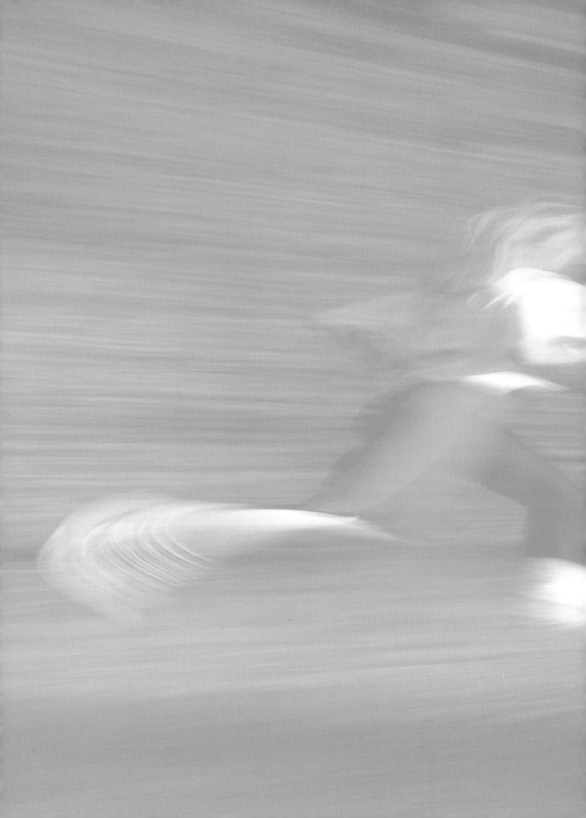

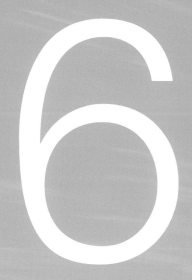

THINKING INTO
COMPETITION

'I let my feet spend as little time on the ground as possible.
From the air, fast down, and from the ground, fast up.'

Jesse Owens

For many people who have taken up running, competition is a natural continuation of their sport. It gives us a chance to see how we measure up against the rest of the crowd. It can be an opportunity to put our training to a serious test. Or it might be the first step on the way to a place in the Olympic team.

Whatever the reason, competition can provide a strong source of motivation and inspire us to greater achievements, both in terms of performance and self-knowledge. It can also be a lot of fun.

There is, however, a potential risk involved for anyone who has worked hard to improve their use. As we have seen, learning to 'inhibit' the unwanted or unnecessary is the first step to making changes. Working in a controlled environment, where stimulation is reduced, reactions can be controlled more easily and use improved. However, when you're out there at the start of a 10-km (6-mile) race, pumped up and raring to go, with lots of other runners bustling around, the environment becomes totally different. Trying to hold on to the memory of good experiences, and a fear of losing them, can lead to a state of paralysis and cause a runner to develop a phobia about 'going wrong'. That's why some would advocate that you should avoid putting yourself in situations where it becomes difficult to inhibit your habitual responses, in order not to compromise your newly developed use. There is plenty to be said for this approach. After all, you can't change and stay the same – alas!

For runners who are already competing but are working to break the negative patterns of tension and strain associated with the activity, a sabbatical from racing is often the only solution. Taking some time away from such a powerful stimulus can enable an athlete to pay attention in a way which is difficult – if not impossible – under competitive conditions.

Is this realistic, though? If you've just got the bug for testing yourself in local 10-km (6-mile) races or you're part of the club squad building up towards the season, how likely are you to back off from that tasty first event on the fixture list because of a concern that you'll sacrifice your carefully developed technique as soon as the starter fires the gun? Here's the common-sense solution. Once you have learned how to think during activity, get out there and apply it. Find the path, stray, and find it again. If you stiffen your neck when you do 200-m (656-ft) repeats, start to figure out a way not to. As you get better at preventing this response, you will run better as well.

I must confess that my perspective on competition is now a little more balanced than it used to be. As someone who has enjoyed pitting his strength, speed and skills against others since childhood, I used to think of a race purely in terms of my time, or whether I could finish ahead of a particular individual. I would get so nervous thatI could barely make it to the starting line. Given the level at which I competed, it all now seems rather silly; but at the time, it was close to being a matter of 'do or die'. Perhaps it is due to the ageing process, but I no longer allow that overpowering need to prove something to have the control over my decision-making that it once had. Instead, the challenge has been to learn to express my 'nature' in ways that don't unduly compromise my use. I now compete much less often than I used to, mostly because I don't want to race if I'm not prepared or, more importantly, if I'm not going to enjoy the experience. And that includes the discomfort which comes from pushing your limits.

A balanced approach

During the Los Angeles Olympics, a number of athletes were asked if they would be willing to take an undetectable drug, which would guarantee them a gold medal but would greatly increase their risk of death within five years. An alarmingly high percentage said they would be willing to do so.

In the book he wrote with his son Sebastian, *Running for Fitness*, Peter Coe discussed the pros and cons of 'the running life'. While running is, for many, a rewarding experience full of joy and learning, for some 'it assumes the proportions of a religion or, worse still, becomes an addiction and an obsession. Its victims become unbalanced and hooked on mileage mania. From there, running can all too easily become a substitute for living and a retreat from the real world. Far from achieving the fitness and sense of well-being that it should bring, it is more likely to end in a frustrating crop of over-use injuries and a lowered level of health from constant over-stress'.

The chief danger with competition is that it can easily cause us to blindly seek the thrill of victory, while overlooking the inherent risks along the way. This, as we have seen, is summed up by the term 'end-gaining'. Trying for too much, too soon, is often a recipe for disaster: in running, as in so many other walks of life, success takes time, patience and discipline.

Greed affects runners as much as it does stockbrokers. I vividly remember how this played out in my first marathon. Fuelled by the vision of breaking the three-hour barrier and the excitement of 15,000 people starting at the same time, I went out with the leaders and coasted through the first mile in just under five minutes. When I tell you that the last mile was completed in slightly over thirteen minutes, including a very fast 'limp finish', you'll get the picture. And, no, I did not break three hours, or even three-and-a-half. It was a very painful lesson, which I only had to repeat two more times before it sank in!

'Everyone loves a winner' is a well-known saying. I like to win. So do most athletes. Unfortunately, winning has been championed by society, and specifically by marketing people in the shoe industry, as the ultimate measure of success in competition. For example, at the Atlanta Olympics, two slogans put out by major

PAULA RADCLIFFE ▼

Alexander Technique teachers who love to comment on Paula Radcliffe's famous 'head bob' should remember that rules which apply to mortals don't necessarily apply to the gods! However, even the best don't always win. Despite meticulous preparation using cutting-edge sports science and technology, Radcliffe was left sobbing on the Athens roadside at the 2004 Olympic Games.

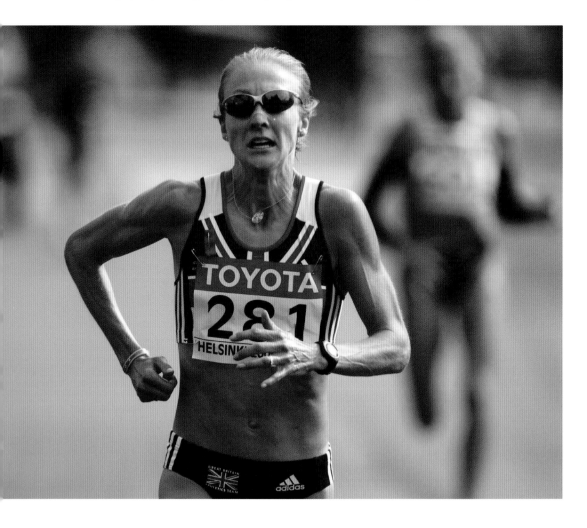

manufacturers were: 'Winning isn't everything, it's the only thing' and 'If you didn't come here for the gold you might as well have stayed home'. These make a complete mockery of the fantastic achievement of just reaching the Olympics.

When you divide the world into winners (good) and losers (bad), it is clear which side most of us want to be on. However, there is only one actual winner in each race – so unless you are exceptionally talented or lucky, you're bound to be disappointed if winning is your only measure of success.

Instead, attempts have been made to redefine competition and winning. 'When runners do their best,' wrote George Sheehan, 'they are all equal. But the paradox is that those far back in the pack exceed the designated winners in the time they must endure the forces that would make them quit. So everyone is a hero. And none are more heroic than those deep in the flow of these struggles against time, distance and self.' Inspiring words, yet small consolation to those who long to be at the front of the pack with the 'real' winners!

Unless, that is, we alter our notions about the purpose of competition and what it means to be a winner. Winning does not always mean that we are the best, or even that we have done our best. You can win without being challenged, or without challenging yourself. You can also cheat in a race and win. However, you can't cheat at what should arguably be the main goal of competition, namely 'to do your best against the rest'.

It's also important to note that unless you fix the outcome of a race, you can't control who wins. Even the best get beaten. Who can forget the sight of Paula Radcliffe sobbing uncontrollably on the Athens roadside, her dream of winning the 2004 Olympic marathon shattered? Britain's greatest-ever female distance runner had prepared meticulously for the big day, drawing on cutting-edge technology and sports science to claim the gold medal that everyone expected would be a formality. Instead, she was undone by Greece's sapping heat and an untimely stomach bug. Trying to control the uncontrollable is a great way to drive yourself nuts, together with everyone around you. So instead, looking at racing and competition through a different lens, we can shift our focus on to those things that are within our power to control, namely ourselves and our reactions. We need to focus on the process of the race, not just the outcome.

Advance preparation

One of the best ways to prepare for a race is to know in advance how you are going to perform. No, this doesn't mean consulting your crystal ball. There are

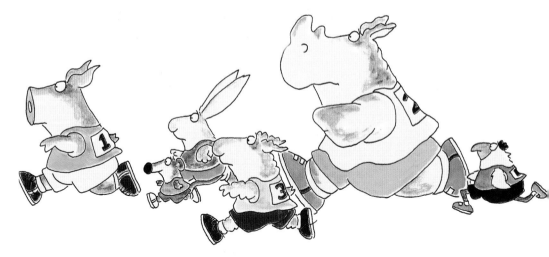

predictive tests which will give you a pretty good idea of how you will perform at your chosen race distance. The better the idea you have, before you start the race, of what your realistic finishing time will be, the greater your success in managing your performance will be. Why is this? Because

Above 'Six is fun for a running race'. It's worth bearing in mind the message of this cartoon and remembering George Sheehan's belief that 'when runners do their best, they are all equal'. Very few of us are able to win all the time, so we must alter our notions of what winning actually means.

when the adrenalin is pumping at the start line, emotion tends to take over – and there is nothing like overstimulated fear reflexes to make both your bladder and your brain run amock. The result? Poor performance.

It is not unrealistic for you to know, barring disaster, what your finishing time in a 5-km (3-mile) race is going to be, to within a minute or so. And yet for many runners, this knowledge and the ability to act on it are complete mysteries. A recent experience comes to mind. I normally have a fairly quick start, but I was left feeling tired and old when a number of runners blew by me as though I was standing still, causing me to worry that my pace judgement had deserted me. I needn't have fretted, though, because within a kilometre their loud breathing and heavy footfalls foretold their fate: a long, hot and painfully slow last 4 km (2½ miles) – a fair way behind me, may I modestly add! This is a classic example of poor race management ('end-gaining' par excellence), witnessed at distances from 400 m to the marathon, and at all levels of competition.

How, then, can you make this type of race the exception rather than the rule? Do your race homework. Back to the 5-km (3-mile) race. One way is to run shorter distances, either as part of a training session or as a time trial. If you can complete 5 x 1 km (0.62 miles) in 4 mins for each kilometre, with a recovery time of 2 mins, this means you can probably expect to complete the entire 5 km (3 miles) in around 21 mins. And you will also have an idea of how fast to run the first kilometre in the race, having practised it frequently in training. So if your split time in the actual race is 3:30, you are either in trouble or your fitness has, for some reason, suddenly made a huge improvement.

If you are the type of runner who likes to go out fast, make this part of your training. Run the first 50 m (164 ft) of every track or fartlek interval hard, in order to train yourself to cope with this kind of demand.

Goal-setting

There is a lot more to goal-setting than just saying to yourself, 'I want to run a marathon or break forty minutes for 10 km (6 miles).' While goal-setting is one of the two most important elements in developing and sustaining your running (the other being a good training partner or group), putting too much emphasis on the goal can rob you of many other reasons to run.

I write this from personal experience: in spite of planning and training really hard for the marathon, with the goal of breaking 2 hrs 50 mins, on the day it was apparent by the third mile that it wasn't going to happen and I quickly readjusted my original splits. At the early stage of the race, it was just taking too much effort to maintain my goal pace. Missing my target initially felt like failure, until I took stock of what I had actually managed to accomplish:

- I had finished a marathon for the first time in twenty-five years.
- I had finished in less than three hours.
- I had finished first in my age category.

From those thoughts came an even deeper sense of satisfaction when I considered what it had taken to achieve that performance:

- I had set a goal and stuck with a training programme through aches and pains.
- I had got out of bed at 6.30 a.m. on a Sunday and run 25 km (15½ miles) at -1°C (still talking to my shrink about that one!).
- I had learnt and implemented a new running technique (the Pose Method).
- I had sustained my form, even when fatigue and discomfort were demanding most of my attention.

● I had kept a sense of humour and perspective when, after the race was over, my car was towed away and my young son dropped the biggest poop in the world and I didn't have a spare nappy.

In hindsight, I can see that the goals were simply targets or markers which helped motivate me and focus my energy. More importantly, they allowed me to experience many rewards which I might otherwise have missed and which stayed with me far longer than the race result.

Jerry Lynch and Warren Scott set out the attributes of what they call the 'warrior runner'. These are worth remembering when trying to set your goals:

The warrior runner:
● Courageously risks failure, learns from setbacks and forges ahead.
● Possesses a multi-dimensional approach to competition.
● Focuses on the process as opposed to the outcome (product).
● Uses a race to gain self-realization.
● Knows her weaknesses and trains to strengthen them.
● Sees competitors as partners who facilitate improvement.
● Understands that racing is a roller-coaster and learns patience to ride the ups and downs.
● Enjoys running for the pleasure it gives.

Jerry Lynch and Warren Scott, *Running Within: A Guide to Mastering the Body-Mind-Spirit Connection*

Preparation on the day

I once had the interesting experience of running a race that finished before I had a chance to catch up. I got lost on the way there and arrived just ten minutes before the start, with nine other athletes to look after. By the time I had changed and handed the athletes their numbers on the starting line, the race was ready to begin. The gun went off and so did I – holding my number scrunched up in my right hand.

During the race, I noticed a number of things. First, I was really pumped up: adrenalin was flowing, mostly from the worry that we wouldn't make it in time to compete. This alone was enough to propel me through the first

HAILE GEBRSELASSIE ▶

Note the gentle spiralling of his torso around a lengthened spine. Gebrselassie also demonstrates the importance of a balanced head, enabling him to look ahead rather than down. His hands are held in a fist, preventing tension there being transmitted to his shoulders.

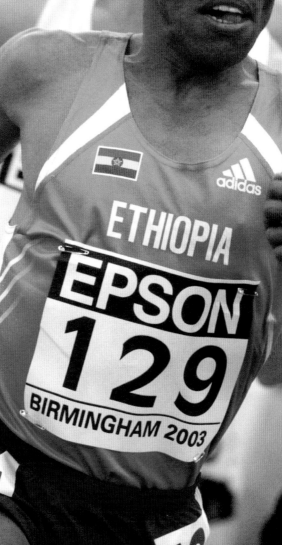

800 m (2,625 ft) in a blind rush: it was simply a matter of 'put it in gear and go'. Although I had run the course before, I kept thinking, 'Oh my goodness, we're at the hill already' or, 'Yes, that was the fast bit where I should speed up', and so on. I kept hoping that something would slow down and let me catch up but, alas, it was me that slowed down and I never caught up.

This experience was a marked contrast from the usual sequence of events when I race. Normally I arrive an hour or so in advance, register and then jog slowly around the course. This gives me a chance to see how the route is set up, note any changes, and plan my race strategy. The strategy would include giving myself mental reminders, such as 'Push the pace here', 'Use my arms more before and after the hill to gain and maintain momentum', 'Take this corner a bit wide so I don't lose speed', 'Shorten my stride through the sandy bit', 'Keep looking ahead', and so on. I would then take time to stretch and do mobility exercises, followed by some accelerations. Each phase of the preparation is designed to bring me (my self) to a state where I am ready to run fast.

The funny thing is that when I go through this kind of detailed rehearsal, the race doesn't seem fast. I have put myself in a position to anticipate, decide and execute rather than simply react. For example, I am not shocked by a hill suddenly appearing 'out of nowhere': I am ready for it and I know what to do. As a result, I am better able to maintain my form and consequently don't slow down as much. I feel as if I have more space and time to be aware of the wider context of the race – spectators, other runners, the weather – and still be able to attend to myself. This allows me to make the many small adjustments that can mean the difference between a good performance and a mediocre one. Most important of all, I have the experience that my whole self is in the race and I am not merely trying to catch up with my legs.

The race: presence

One of the interesting things about competition is what you can learn about yourself, and how you react in stressful situations. How well do you maintain, for example, your poise (that is, the integrity of the head-neck-back relationship)? Your clarity of intention? Your sense of perspective when you are overwhelmed by pre-race jitters? Your ability to maintain your grace under pressure? Reacting correctly in the heat of the race requires us to have presence, a quality that is directly related to the way that we use ourselves. It requires us to take advantage of that little space between stimulus and response: choice flavoured with clarity of intention, intelligence, courage and awareness can play a liberating role for the competitive runner.

Peter Coe once told an interesting story about his son's failure to win the gold medal for the 800 m at the 1980 Moscow Olympics. Coe was the odds-on favourite for victory. He was the world record holder, in excellent shape, and was considered invincible over the distance. As with Radcliffe twenty-four years later, the pressure on him to win was enormous. Coe Senior recounted that his son seemed rather withdrawn on the morning of the race, quieter than usual. He did not comment on it at the time, because his style was to give an athlete enough room to run his own race. But he now knows that on this occasion it was a mistake. Coe's 'head was not in the race', and by the time he woke up, another great British athlete, Steve Ovett, had

SEBASTIAN COE ▼

After failing to win the 800 m gold medal at the Moscow Olympics when his 'head was not in the race', Sebastian Coe regained and maintained his focus to beat favourite Steve Ovett in the 1500 m final.

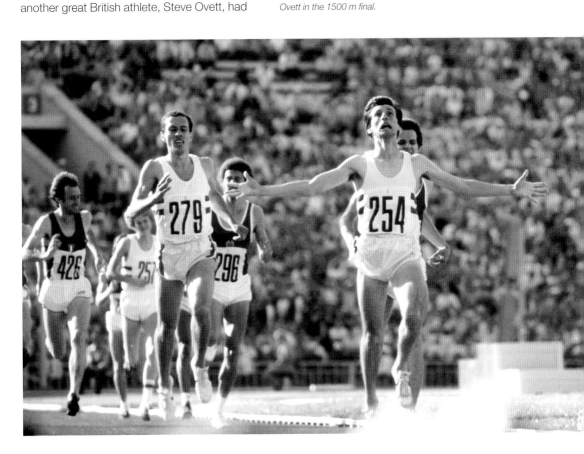

CASE STUDY
A runner's experience: Andrew

I have started to make a distinction between practising and training. I now include one or two sessions each week of drills – though I do get strange looks when people see me jumping from one leg to the other while my ankles are attached to a tree by a rubber tube!

I try to focus on four things:

- Keeping my ankles soft when my feet land;
- Falling;
- Pulling up my ankle underneath my bottom;
- Swinging my arms loosely from the shoulder.

Of the four, I am worst at keeping the ankles soft. I often seem to have tightness on the outside of the lower leg and into the ankle joint. Sometimes the joint itself becomes painful, though the pain always goes away once the ankle is properly warmed up. It can take a lot of ankle rotations, however.

One of the most interesting lessons for me was when I was in a 5,000 m track race – my first race after spending a week on a Pose Method course. With 1,000 m (0.62 miles) to go, I thought: 'Right, this is it, the business end of the race. Up the tempo and run hard until you catch that guy in front.' As I tried to run harder, my breathing became more laboured and my shoulders rose closer and closer to my ears. And the guy in front didn't get any nearer. Suddenly, I said to myself, 'What are you doing? You spend all week on that course learning to run and the first race you get into you forget everything you learnt!' So I relaxed, dropped my shoulders and focused on just pulling my legs from the ground. Very soon, the guy in front became the guy behind and I went on to record a season's best.

too much of a lead for Seb to make up. He was not close enough at the finish for his tremendous kick to have any impact and, in spite of an incredible effort, he finished second. For many people this would have been a great performance, but for Coe it was considered a disastrous failure.

I work with a lot of musicians. I have noticed that when musicians perform in public, they sometimes try and escape from their anxiety by disconnecting or hiding from the outside world. You can see it in their eyes: they aren't all there. Rather than focusing on what lies ahead, all they want to do is get the hell out of the place. The effect is that there is a difference in the quality of their performance. This is particularly true for singers, who have nowhere to hide. When this happens in an Olympic final, perhaps as a way of coping with the incredible pressure and expectation, the result is a lack of availability to respond appropriately to the situation at hand. In Coe's case, by the time he had reconnected, the damage had been done.

There is a second part to this story. Peter Coe recalls that he went against his custom when it came to the final of the 1,500 m, and he gave Seb some rather direct advice about staying with the pace. He said something along the lines of, 'You stick so close to so-and-so that if he goes to the loo, you'll be in there handing him the paper!' The upshot was that the overwhelming favourite to win the 1,500 m, Steve Ovett, was beaten by Seb Coe – who did not lose his focus and was therefore in a position to use his kick to great effect.

The race: avoiding distractions

In the final of the 100 m at the 1999 World Championships, the great Canadian sprinter Bruny Surin made a tremendous start and was leading the field at the halfway mark. But at this point, Surin said afterwards, he panicked and tightened, perhaps in surprise at finding himself in such a favourable position, and then tried to accelerate.

The cost of such a tiny distraction in world-class sprinting can be very high, given that the difference between the top competitors is mere tenths of a second. His coach, Michel Portmann, was watching the race from the sidelines and saw Surin's head pull back at this point. The world record holder, America's Maurice Greene, was then able to pass him and reach the line first. According to Portmann, there was no need for Surin to accelerate at that point; he simply needed to maintain his rhythm and let the rest of the field try and catch him. Instead, he started to worry about winning. It was his momentary focus on this idea, rather than staying with 'the plan', that caused his downfall. He needed to forget about winning, yet continue to do the things that would allow him to win – no small order under the circumstances.

Sprinters are taught to visualize their lane as a tunnel, in order to help shut out the potential distractions of rivals, officials and the crowd. The problem for Surin was that when something did intrude into the imaginary tunnel, his reaction was similar to the 'startle response' (a reflexive reaction to a sudden loud noise). This disrupted his focus and rhythm, and made him try to correct his reaction by accelerating, which then disturbed his coordination.

Staying focused

When I was competing at 800 m, I remember my coach saying that if your attention lapses, it takes the best part of 60 m (197 ft) to refocus. It is amazing to think that in a race of such intensity my mind could wander, but it did. And I can recall how much harder it was to literally get back on track than on those occasions when I kept my focus. There is a Zen saying: 'When chopping wood and carrying water, just chop wood and carry water.' This implies that the goal when running and racing is not to escape from what you're engaged in, but to

JUSTIN GATLIN & MAURICE GREENE ▶
Two world and Olympic champions, Justin Gatlin and Maurice Greene, completely 'in the moment'. Sprinters are taught to visualise their lane as a tunnel in order to shut out the potential distractions of rivals, officials and the crowd. The cost of a tiny loss of focus can be very high, given that races are decided by mere tenths of a second.

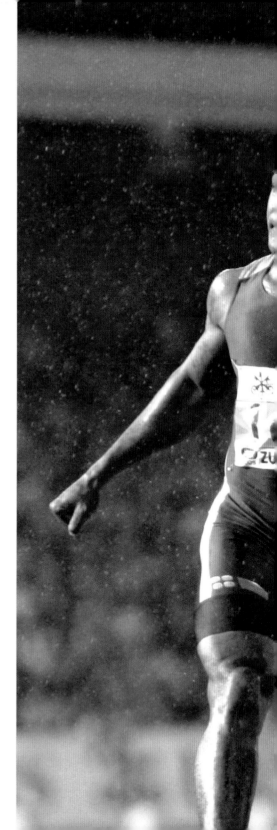

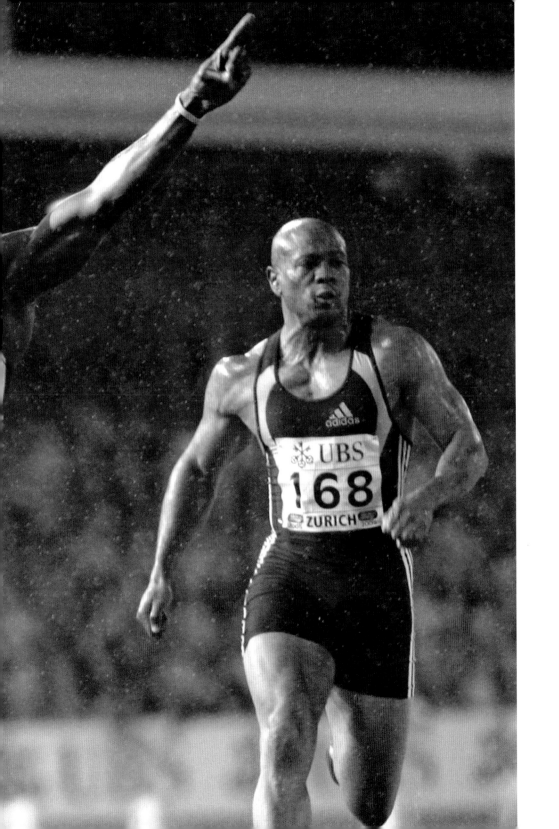

embrace it – to 'just run'. Trying to force oneself into a state of 'concentration' is ineffective and wastes energy that could be more gainfully employed to run better.

It helps to develop a series of short-term goals as a way of more fully engaging oneself with the process. In the aforementioned 800 m, I would divide the race into eight 100-m (328-ft) sections, each with its own specific requirements. For the first section, my goal was to accelerate aggressively to near maximum speed around the first curve, to avoid getting entangled with other runners. Within those parameters I paid attention to my form, staying free in the shoulders and not holding my breath, as was my tendency under these circumstances. So there were always two levels of awareness occurring simultaneously: what I intended to do and the way I was doing it. If there was too much outer focus, I might come out of the turn tight and in severe oxygen debt. If there was too much inner focus, I could be knocked off course by a rival.

By the last 40 m (131 ft) of the first 100 m (328 ft), I would begin anticipating the requirements for the next section – or risk being halfway through it before waking up. Anticipation is the key to smooth transitions and to maintaining focus, otherwise you risk being surprised and performing a variation of the startle reflex.

Perhaps the most critical transition in an 800-m race is coming out of the final turn, when fatigue and lactic acid are combining to leave you breakdancing down the home stretch. If you haven't thought about keeping your length, releasing tension in your shoulders and staying smooth before this point, you may find those last few metres a real struggle – and the difference between winning and finishing down the field.

The same kind of system can be used in races of longer duration. Here are some ideas to help you maintain or regain focus and avoid distraction:

Count your steps

Cadence or stride frequency is an important component of good running. Checking to see if you are maintaining a cadence above 180 steps per minute is a great way to bring yourself 'back to the moment'. Simply count the number of times your right (or left) foot touches the ground for one minute. I like to count in groups of ten as I find it easier not to get lost! If you're 'in the zone', your right foot should touch the ground (lightly, we hope), around ninety times or more during that one-minute period. When you find yourself becoming obsessed with extraneous ideas such as pain and discomfort, winning or your finishing time, simply go back to counting steps.

Synchronize your breathing

Explore the connection between your breathing rhythm and your cadence. You will be breathing in for a certain number of steps and then out for a certain number. When I am running at race speed, I tend to breathe in for two steps and out for the same number (2-2). When I am running at a more comfortable pace, the rhythm is more like 4-4. Sometimes it is uneven, as when I am trying to breathe out for longer than I breathe in as a way of calming myself down. I know that if I am at a 1-1 rhythm, I am not going to last very long at that pace and therefore try not to go there before the home stretch. By the same token, a 3-3 or 4-4 breathing pattern means that I could be running more quickly.

Look ahead

Runners tend to look down or, when looking ahead, tend not to see what they are looking at. Finding a 'target' about 100 m (328 ft) down the road and focusing on it as you run is a great way to stay present. But when you find yourself looking at the next telegraph pole and not really seeing it, pick out some detail and try to describe it to yourself or an imaginary friend as a way of stopping your mind wandering. In a race, I find the idea of keeping a connection with the runner in front of me, even imagining a string stretched between us pulling me along, helps me maintain a more even pace when I begin to tire or lose focus.

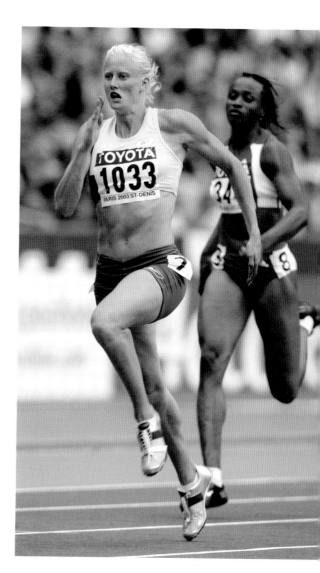

CAROLINE KLUFT ▶

What's not to like about this great athlete? Here she is making the kind of powerful effort that takes her into the 'up'. Her head is balanced, her eyes are looking ahead and her arms are used with immense efficiency – all while she is dealing with the demands of a highly competitive race.

CASE STUDY
A runner's experience: Patrick

When I moved to South Africa in 1998, I saw it as a great chance to get back into shape and try to improve my time over 5 km (3 miles) and 10 km (6 miles). I had been living in northern Canada for three years, where the climate was not conducive to any form of regular training. I joined the Witbank Road Runners' Club and soon found that the recreational running scene in South Africa was huge, but almost solely focused on two races – the Two Oceans Marathon (56 km/ 35 miles) in Cape Town and the Comrades Marathon (90 km/56 miles) between Pietermaritzburg and Durban. With no middle-distance training partners and constant pressure from my running club friends, I started to train for these two ultra marathons.

Having never raced more than 12 km (7½ miles), and my focus at university being the 800 m and 1,500 m, I slowly started the mileage build-up that was required. I had used the Alexander Technique all through my university career to mitigate (and eventually eliminate) the constant back pain that I lived with in my early years of running, and continued to use it throughout my eight months of training.

I ran my first marathon in February 1999, which qualified me for the Two Oceans in April and for the Comrades in June. My target time for the Comrades was 7 hrs 30 mins, the cut-off for a silver medal, requiring an average of 5 mins per kilometre.

As the races approached, a typical week of training was as follows. Monday: 15 km (9 miles); Tuesday: 8-km (5-mile) time trial; Wednesday: 21 km (13 miles); Thursday: 10 km (6 miles); Friday: 8 km (5 miles); Saturday: 32 km (20 miles); Sunday: 15 km (9 miles).

The Two Oceans Marathon is the most beautiful route I have ever run. It follows the seaside roads through Cape Town and shows the city at its best. However, the last 14 km (8½ miles) were not fun as I suffered calf and hamstring cramps, finishing in a time of 4 hrs 29 mins.

As I continued towards the Comrades Marathon, I used the semi-supine position [see Chapter 5] on a daily basis to ensure that my back and neck would not break down under the heavy training schedule. A week before the race, I sat down with two experienced Comrades runners and planned my strategy: split in 3 hrs 45 mins and hold on.

As the race started, I felt good and ran comfortably through the marathon mark. I then walked through my first water station at about 50 km (31 miles) to take the aspirin that had been recommended to dull the pain. The Comrades Marathon alternates the direction between Pietermaritzburg and Durban each year, creating an uphill race and a downhill race. In 1999, it was downhill, ending at the coast in Durban. I initially thought this would help, as the first 50 km (31 miles) or so were in the undulating hills as you approach the ocean, with the last 40 km (25 miles) dropping approximately 800 m (2,625 ft) in altitude. As I started the first of the long descents, my legs again started to cramp. When I saw the next distance marker showing I had 33 km (20½ miles) to go, I knew it was going to be a long day. I found myself focusing on small goals, such as 'Run to that tree'. If I got there without cramping, I would run to the next.

The long descents put constant pressure on my quads and hamstrings. I was reduced to running until I suffered cramp, then would walk until it stopped. When I finally saw King's Park where the raced finished, I found myself obsessed with avoiding walking in front of the 15,000 spectators who had gathered at the finish line. I walked for the two lamp-posts in front of the stadium, then ran in. I crossed the line in 8 hrs 47 mins – a time that I will never forget.

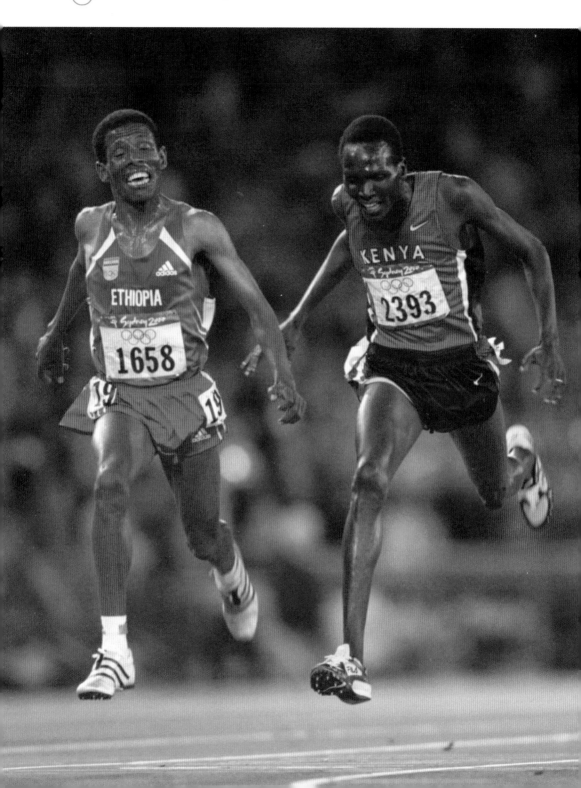

Check your form

As you tire, it is easy to lose form and pay a higher price for your efforts than you need to. While the middle of a race is not the time to get too clever with your form, it is worth monitoring some of the little things that can make such a difference to your overall performance. For example, releasing tension in both the thumbs and the armpits can greatly reduce shoulder rigidity and its negative effect on arm movement. Heavy, loud footsteps are also a bad sign, and it may be necessary to renew your upward direction. In fact, doing so regularly will help prevent you from pounding the ground. Develop a checklist of key form points and refer to them regularly when competing, to help you maintain a balance between where you are going and how you are getting there.

Progression

When runners first start competing, they sometimes go through a wonderful period where races bring a stream of personal-best (PB) performances. This is instant reward for the effort expended. Alas, it soon passes, and the reward of a personal best becomes more and more difficult to achieve.

When improvement becomes rarer, many runners become disillusioned and quit. They haven't learned, as George Leonard puts it in his book *The Ultimate Athlete*, 'to love the plateau'. As a coach, I try to encourage my athletes to stick with the programme. In other words, they must believe that following the training schedule will enable them to reach their goals. Yet some runners find it very difficult to hang in there day after day, allowing time for the adaptations that training produces to take place. They suffer from what I call a 'High School mentality'.

In Canada every May or June, near the end of the academic year, many High Schools have a track and field meeting. Runners prepare for this event for two or three weeks and, on the big day, those with the most natural athletic talent win all the medals and get all the glory. This masks the real requirements for developing their potential. Arriving at university, the next step up (where everyone has talent) requires a commitment to train for eleven months of the year. The sacrifices needed to be competitive at this level come as a shock to the system. A parallel scenario for British runners is the difference between being a star at schools level and making the step up to county or inter-club league competitions.

◀ **HAILE GEBRSELASSIE & PAUL TERGAT**

This thrilling battle between two of the world's greatest ever athletes shows the importance of maintaining focus right to the finish line. Both men may have planned the race by dividing it into a series of short-term goals, each anticipating the requirements of the next section. The key for all runners is to avoid the risk of being surprised.

On track

Training and competing on the track rather than running on the road is a bit like swimming in a pool compared to the open water. On the track, you know exactly how fast you are going, and there's no escape from the tyranny of the stopwatch. Also, the route is fairly predictable – you run straight and turn left occasionally!

I've trained and competed on the track for more than twenty years and for the most part have loved it. 'Boring', some of you might say. Yes and no. It's funny, when you are in the middle of a workout or a race, how the external scenery disappears. During my first marathon, I passed the Niagara Falls and didn't see or hear anything! I like the familiarity and the rhythm of running on the track. It provides an uncompromising and unrelenting reality check. Do you think you can run at such and such a pace? Get out on a track and see. I remember training at a track alongside a runner who never tired of recounting his fantastic performances in various road races. We were all impressed, but soon became sceptical when his track performance was not even close to what he claimed to have run on the road. Another example of the 'short-course PB'!

Personal bests

The personal best is the measure of our quest to achieve our potential. Approached with balance and perspective, trying to set a new PB can be an exhilarating and life-affirming experience, demanding courage and focused effort. Training yourself to try and go further or faster than ever before is, in one sense, what racing is all about and what competition can help you achieve.

The irony for me was that I often achieved my best performances when I didn't care about them. It wasn't a matter of just showing up at a race and saying 'Oh, I think I'll set a PB today.' There were months of training and preparation involved. It was just that I'd let go of 'having to set the record' and focused instead on smaller, achievable targets: staying smooth, not getting too excited, aiming for the next checkpoint, coping with discomfort, and so on. When it all came together on the day, the PB just 'did itself'. The interesting thing, now that I'm in my fifties and the possibility of setting a new PB is sadly behind me, is that when I compete with the same qualities, the same focus, the same enthusiasm and courage, even though my times are slower, the sense of accomplishment is still there.

HAILE GEBRSELASSIE ▶

For athletes of Gebrselassie's calibre, there is money to be made by the pursuit of records. For we lesser mortals, the pursuit of a 'personal best' can be an exhilarating and life-affirming experience, demanding courage and focused effort. Training to go faster or further than before is what competition can help us achieve. However, it needs to be tackled with balance and perspective.

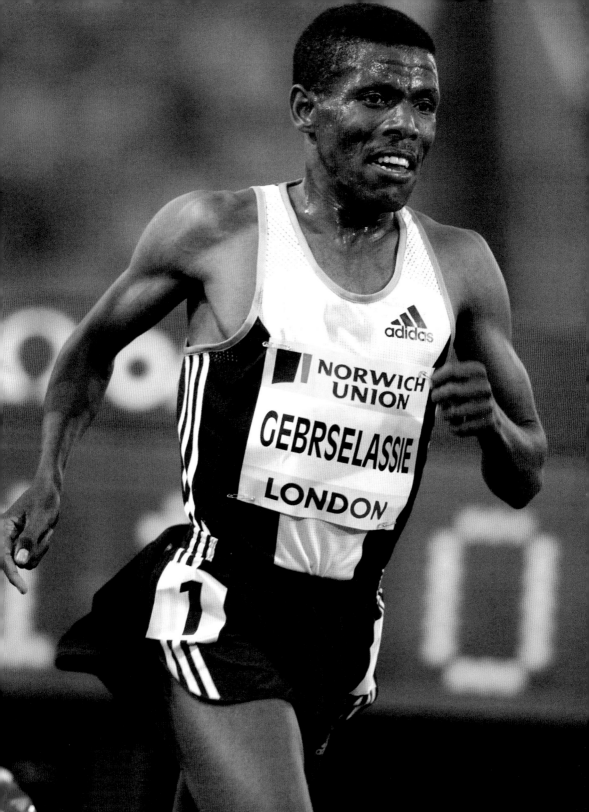

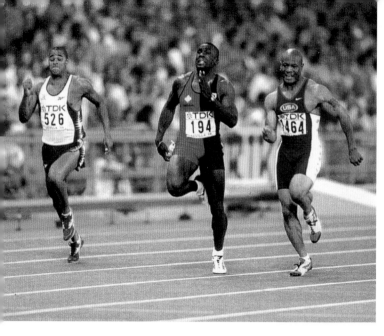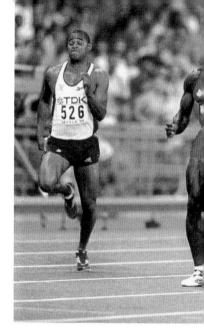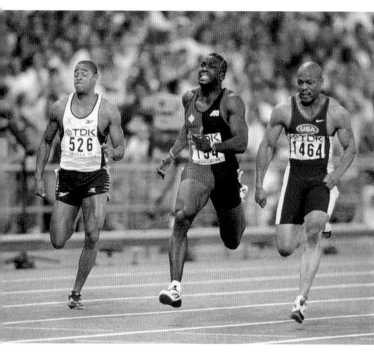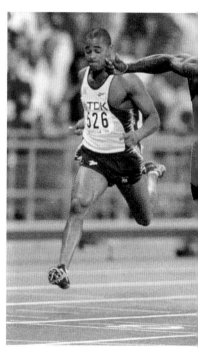

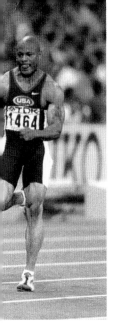
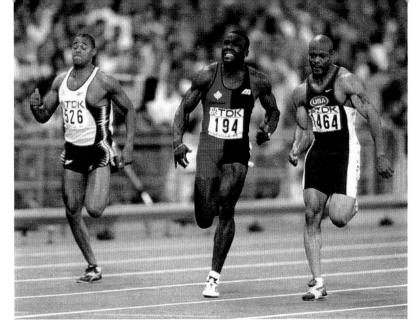
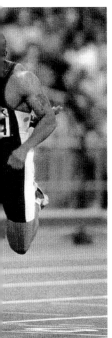
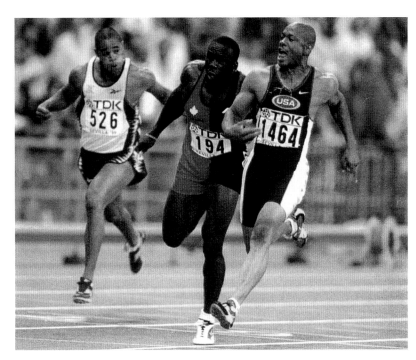

BRUNY SURIN ▲

This sequence of photographs shows how Surin (number 194) lost the chance of a gold medal in the 100 m at the 1999 World Championships. Unexpectedly ahead of the field at the halfway mark, he panicked and tightened. Instead of maintaining his rhythm and letting the others try to catch him, he started to 'worry about winning'.

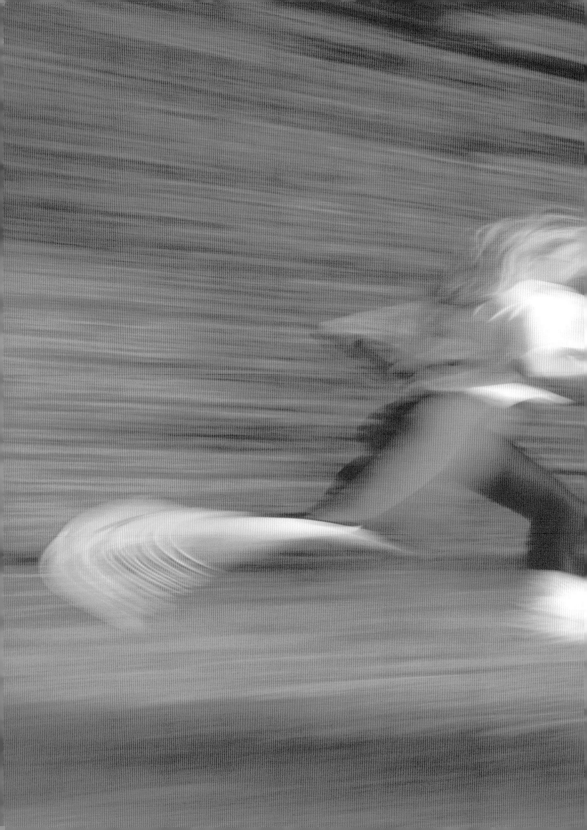

7

INJURIES – AND HOW TO AVOID THEM

'To urge competitiveness and to urge caution in quick succession is not a contradiction. The longer you keep running well, the longer you will stay well. And if you are running for fitness, anything that curtails your running also curtails your fitness. But lasting success has never been achieved without understanding the need for moderation. When applying increasing doses of stress – for that is what a large part of race training is – giving the correct opportunities for recovery requires careful thought. And if the top performers can practise restraint in their training build-up, then so can fitness runners, for certainly the same pressures are not on them.'

Peter and Sebastian Coe

Injured runners are as common as wasps around a bowl of strawberries. In *The New Competitive Runner's Handbook*, Bob Glover states: 'Like other athletes, competitive runners must learn to accept the inevitability of injury and illness. It is safe to say that every year of competitive running will find you injured or ill at least a few times.' The reality of this statement is echoed by another well-known runner/author, Jeff Galloway, who reckons that in his twenty-five-year career he suffered more than a hundred lay-offs.

As a marathoner in the late 1970s, I suffered a wide variety of injuries and found myself constantly climbing out of the valley of rehabilitation. Looking back on that period now, I can't remember a time when I wasn't nursing a physical problem of some kind, in addition to the colds and flu that always seem to attack competitive athletes. Imagine my surprise when, after I began training as an Alexander Technique teacher in 1981, I no longer seemed to get hurt. In fact, from 1982 to 1999 (when I pulled a groin muscle trying to be a sprinter!), I did not suffer a single injury in spite of training for and competing in the 800 m and 1,500 m. I'm not talking about the little niggles and aches that accompany any hard physical effort, but the kind of problem that involves time away from the track, physiotherapy or some other treatment, and a period of rebuilding.

This was not because I was babying myself. I was still doing workouts that pulled no punches. So what was making the difference?

There is a Zen saying: 'When the pupil is ready, the teacher arrives'. One day on the track, quite by chance (or so it seemed), I met a coach who told me I needed to learn how to run. I was both insulted and intrigued. What the hell was he on about? I'd finished five marathons and clocked up thousands of miles – I knew how to run. In fact, I had developed an ultra-efficient marathon shuffle, with a pronounced heel strike, tight arms, and a tendency to sit on my legs. It didn't feel like that, of course, but when I saw myself on video, I was shocked. He was right: there was room for improvement. The seed had been planted and I knew that, in order to get faster, my form required a major overhaul.

Did I make a connection between running form and injuries at the time? Absolutely not. Initially, it was all about learning to run faster. It was only later that I realized this was an important step towards injury-free running. In hindsight I think that, like many, I had assumed running was a natural activity. It was simply a matter of buying a good pair of shoes and getting in shape: I had been a pretty decent ice hockey player so becoming a runner was simply a matter of putting in the practice. I never considered that running might be 'natural' for Ethiopians or

Kenyans because that was how they got to school or visited their neighbours. My basic modes of transport were bike, bus or car.

Why is this important? Consider the following. Biomechanical research indicates that in running, impact forces are three to five times greater than in walking. An average runner will take between 150–200 steps per minute. For someone who completes a marathon in 3 hrs 20 mins at a rate of 160 strides per minute, this adds up to more than 32,000 impacts. Add the hundreds of training kilometres and a burning ambition to break the three-hour barrier, and you have a recipe for disaster.

During my training as an Alexander Technique teacher, I became extremely keen to prevent a recurrence of the many problems that had plagued my running. One of the few things I was capable of doing in the early stages of the course was to observe what I was doing to myself when I ran. Not only did this make running more interesting, but it meant that I was beginning to spot potential issues. In addition, where before I had been mainly concerned with how far, how fast and how often, my mental checklist now included how easy, how free and how smooth.

There is, however, one key issue to deal with here: the fact that many runners are irrational zealots. For some, it is a badge of honour that they train when stressed and tired, and compete while injured. For competitive club runners, loyalty to the team can override all thoughts of personal health and well-being. Former European and Commonwealth marathon gold medallist Ron Hill has, famously, run every day since 1964 – even though he suffered a car crash in 1993 and broke his sternum, he still managed to run a mile the next day. A friend ran for charity while suffering from achilles tendonitis, which was severe enough to require his leg to be encased in plaster for more than a week when it was over. Paula Radcliffe admits in her autobiography: 'If a physio tells me to try a run and that a little bit of awareness of an injury is fine but when it gets to pain I must stop, I find it very difficult. For me it's very hard to work out where awareness crosses the line into pain.' There are similar examples everywhere.

As for me, I often trained when I was injured, didn't take enough time for rest, ran in -35°C weather, and so on – all to break three hours for the marathon. When viewed from a distance this looks crazy, but at the time it seemed perfectly normal – in fact, it was more the rule than the exception. I recently worked with a man in his early forties, who had run a half-marathon in 72 mins when in his thirties but was no longer able to run at all because of severe sciatica. He told me that of the twelve athletes he trained with in his twenties and thirties, none was still running: injuries had claimed them all. I have no doubt that I would be in the same position had I not stopped to reassess what I was doing and why, and decided on a different course of action.

Use and running mechanics

Good mechanics help reduce the strain that competitive running places on the body; after all, the stresses that exist for the casual runner are multiplied many times for the racer. While the fun runner can choose to miss a race, the club athlete may find it much harder to miss a training session or a competition, since coaches and team-mates may be counting on her.

Above club runners are the elite athletes, capable of weekly mileages that would leave the rest of us heading for the local casualty department. There is an understandable temptation to think that by copying their schedules, we too can improve our performances. But the life of an elite athlete is very different from that of the average runner. As Paula Radcliffe describes, 'Much of my adult life has been consumed by running, resting, racing and recovering.' Very few elite

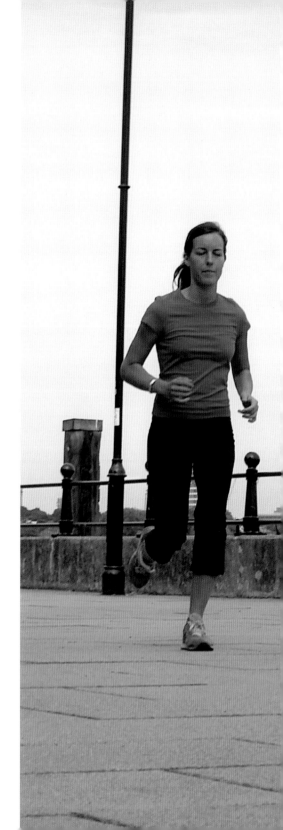

Right Impact forces in running are three to five times greater than in walking. Coupled with the fact that a marathon can demand more than 32,000 impacts, the need to pay constant attention to use is obvious.

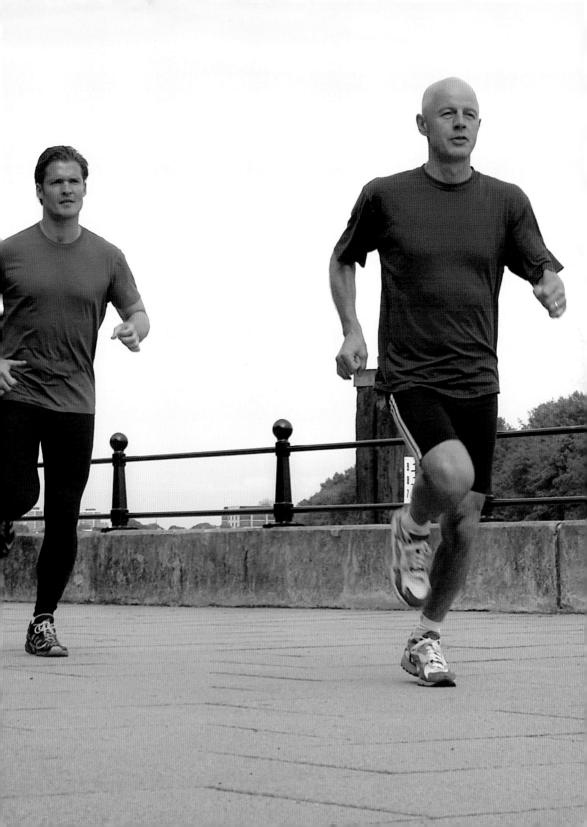

athletes have to get the kids off to school in the morning, put in a full day at the office, take their daughter to ballet class, repair the garden fence, cook the evening meal – and then find a few spare moments for a quality training session. It's this kind of hectic schedule, where there is simply no time for the luxury of resting and recovering, that leads to injury.

Instead, the intelligent runner can reduce the risk of injury by keeping her total mileage down. As a guide, the total weekly mileage for a novice runner should be about double the length of her longest run. For example, in a week when your longest run is 25 km (15½ miles), your total mileage should be no more than 50 km (31 miles). More advanced runners will aim for a higher weekly total but this should never be more than triple the length of the long run (75 km/46½ miles, if your longest run is 25 km/15½ miles). Running more than this can bring on symptoms of over-training.

Aim to increase the intensity of those quality workouts. This will also increase the risk and potential cost of bad form or misdirected effort. But, as the level of competition gets tougher, so does the potential price one has to pay to stay in the game.

Over-training and under-recovery

Regular exercise builds strength and stamina, helps to keep you well balanced temperamentally, promotes a regular sleeping pattern and generally makes you feel good about yourself. Excessive exercise reverses all these trends.

The easiest way to tell if you are overdoing it is to decide whether you feel unnaturally tired. Are you dragging yourself out for a run and feeling lethargic while you're doing it – or even when you're resting? Are you moody and irritable? Depressed and anxious? Suffering from decreased appetite and weight loss, nausea and an upset stomach? Have you got persistent soreness in your muscles and joints? Are you falling prey to colds and viral illnesses?

When you ask your body to do more than it realistically can, you run the risk of over-training. This may consist of too many long runs in a week. Or too many intense training sessions. Or of simply not listening to your body when it tells you to slow down and take a rest. It's important to decide whether the fatigue is caused by over-training or by under-recovery. Short periods of fatigue are an inevitable part of the training process. It's when there is an accumulation of fatigue, which is not dealt with by adequate recovery, that you can begin to suffer from under-performance.

How to avoid over-training and under-recovery

Listen to your body

After a run, you should feel better, not worse. If your body responds by sending you signals of pain and fatigue, stop, rest and rethink your routine.

Allow plenty of rest

It is inadvisable for all but the most experienced competitive athletes to run every day. If you push your body too hard and too often, you risk wearing it down.

Drink water regularly

Drink at least 2 litres (3½ pints) per day. This is especially important during exercise. Water makes up 60 per cent of your body weight and 70 per cent of your muscle tissue. If you do not restore your fluid levels, you risk fatigue and overheating.

Eat well

While exercising, you use energy that has been stored as carbohydrate and fat. You need to replenish these stores or your body will naturally slow down. Make sure you eat complex carbohydrates such as pasta and cereal, plenty of fruit and vegetables, plus adequate protein (whether from meat or another source).

Go easy on the painkillers

Pain is a sign that your body has a problem. Using medicine to mask pain is likely to cause more serious damage.

Vary your training schedule

You may be driving yourself too hard because you are bored. Make sure every run or workout is stimulating. Cross-training is just as important for runners as it is for other sportspeople.

Keep a training log

As well as recording how far you ran and for how long, include more subjective material. Did you sleep well the previous night? How did the run feel? Was it stimulating? Did you finish with a sense of achievement – or relief? This is potentially the best of the monitoring tools for detecting over-training.

A runner's experience: Neil

It has long been one of my bugbears that (in English schools at least) you're rarely actually taught any sport. That's to say the fundamentals – the pure techniques and theories – are seemingly only built on when a natural flair is spotted. Boring as the basics may be, in the light of my 'Art of Running' experiences it has become increasingly obvious that I developed some bad habits early on.

I always thought running was such a fundamental attribute that unless you were an elite athlete, running style was something you had as a birthright – as personal to you as a fingerprint and equally unchangeable. How wrong could I be?

At school I was a little-above-average sportsman and, as I suspect happens to many people, my fitness levels went through the floor on entering college. It wasn't until I'd got a job that I began playing football again. Sunday morning leagues are not noted for their peak physical specimens and deft footwork, but I figured it was as good a place as any to begin regaining some fitness.

After my second season (and ironically in a training session) I turned awkwardly, felt my knee pop and hit the ground like a sack of potatoes. Having never suffered a serious injury before, I thought I was invincible. I tried in vain to get back on the pitch the following season, but every tackle saw my knee collapse. I knew I'd done something irreversible but it took an arthroscopy to reveal that I had snapped the anterior cruciate ligament (ACL) in my right knee.

The injury and operation left me without a fitness outlet. My physio advised that I should find a gym and get a good rehab programme. To do any active work with that joint I'd need to radically improve the stability around the damaged knee. Up to that time, I'd always been wary of gyms. Now I had little choice but to join one. And there came my next shock.

I watched and learned that most of the posing and grunting was done by people with the worst form. For the first time, I realized that poor technique was the fast track to injuries. I began to focus on regaining my general fitness, with the emphasis on leg strength, and discovered that running was the activity I found most rewarding. During my first hesitant steps on the treadmill, I couldn't imagine how it was possible to run with bad technique. I'll never forget those first few paces. As I remembered what it was like to pick up pace, I couldn't help breaking into a spontaneous grin.

Gradually, I began to take things a little more seriously. I carried on running in the gym, with occasional forays on the roads and grass wherever possible. I began to set my sights on running 10 km (6 miles) in under forty minutes. I knew I could reach the required fitness so long as my limbs stayed intact. But that was the problem – I was getting constant problems with calf tears. I assumed that other muscles were compensating for the instability in my knee and getting overworked.

For a number of years, I fought the injuries with periods of rest, rebuilding and intermittent spells of physiotherapy. Then I came across an advert for Malcolm Balk's workshops. As a designer, 'The Art of Running' appealed to me on an aesthetic level. Surely, here was the reason elite runners look so good while in motion: form follows function. As I looked more closely, I discovered that aesthetics had nothing to do with it. However, the workshop did promise to make my running more efficient – and quite possibly shed light on the reasons why I was repeating these injuries.

Typically, fate intervened again twenty-four hours before the workshop, when my knee popped out while I was doing some DIY. More surgery and rehab followed. I was now minus an ACL and about a third of my stabilizing cartilage on the same leg! Unable to do any impact work and keen to use the time profitably, I took the opportunity to learn to swim. Properly. Swimming was another sport that I thought you had to have a natural aptitude to enjoy – and I was certainly no water baby.

Concentrating on body alignment and relaxation, I began to learn that technique triumphs over effort. I realized that if I could do this in water, my studious approach to technique would reap rewards on land.

I finally managed to get to see Malcolm. It was the video footage he took which proved the most revelatory. It showed that I was running with an anterior tilt to my pelvis – or, as my girlfriend put it more succinctly, 'You run with your bottom sticking out.' It clearly showed that all my forward motion was coming from my quads and calves as I tried to push the ground backwards. My toe-off showed that I was contracting muscles and springing upwards, not forwards.

On recovery, the first part of my foot to hit the ground was the heel. The heel strike indicated that I was leading with my foot and, because it was landing a reasonable distance in front of my body, I was effectively braking any forward momentum. Extension, contraction and impact – no wonder my calves were paying for all the stress. On top of all this, my upper body was as tightly strung as a concert piano.

Malcolm first taught me to run tall and to be balanced. The next big leap (or rather, short hop) was learning to use the hamstrings to lift a relaxed lower leg up and under the body. It was about here that I feared the pain would start – all that weight on one remaining leg, and what about the impact when the foot returned to earth? How was my knee going to cope? I was just waiting to feel the scars opening again.

In fact, it proved to be eminently more comfortable than my regular running style. It showed me that I was actually expending energy putting the foot down when all I needed to do was let it fall, relaxed, on to the ball of the foot. When the head/body is balanced correctly (on a slightly bent leg), and everything else is relaxed and loose, there is naturally less tension to cause the stress tears.

Once I'd got the knack of static hops I found it a great deal easier to lift and remain balanced than pushing off and up from the toes.

Next, we went into motion. Slowly at first, finding that the hops naturally took you forwards. Then quicker, trying to use only gravity to assist a slight shift forward in the body's centre of gravity, to increase speed. That's when the sensation of running on the legs and not with them really hit home – a revelation. And all of this without a twinge in either knees or calves.

My injuries forced me into a different way of thinking about fitness. Time spent considering technique is helping me to overcome the hurdles and I'm now able to appreciate the process as well as the product. I know I have a way to go to get that sub-40-minute 10 km (6 miles) and, as you can tell, I've not yet lost that end-gaining fixation. But what I will no longer do is substitute effort for technique.

HOW TO RUN WELL (AND AVOID RUNNING BADLY)

Athletes, coaches and sports psychologists often use the phrase 'getting in the zone'. It refers to the quest for those fleeting moments when everything comes together and we are able to perform at our very best, with little or no gap between intention and actualization.

When Sebastian Coe set a new world record for 800 m, he described his performance in these terms. He is not the only athlete to speak in near-mystical, Zen-like language of this 'peak experience'. As a result, runners often resort to various rituals in the hope of maintaining or rediscovering this elusive state of grace. Throughout this book, we've explored ways to 'think in activity' – the more we practise doing so, the less elusive 'the zone' may become.

How, then, do we capture peak experience? We have seen that we can't always rely on our instincts to guide us correctly or accurately in our activities. Part of the reason for this is the fact that many of us do not have a clear idea of how to do something – of what is required and, more importantly, what isn't.

Take, for example, the way that most people sit down. They begin by shortening the neck and pulling the head back, which compresses the spine. Finally, they aim their bottom towards the chair, causing the lower back to stiffen and arch. Then they drop their weight – in other words, collapse – into the chair.

Why? Common responses include: 'I'm afraid the chair won't be there' or 'I'm trying to keep my balance'. In fact, most of us have forgotten (if we ever really knew) what is needed to sit. Instead, we rely on a conception that is built from our experience. We need to replace this with something that is much more free and unobstructed, and which respects the way we are actually designed to bend – along the lines of the head, leading the spine into length, while the knees release out over the toes. This enables you to sit in a chair by expending minimal effort. To see natural, undistorted movement, watch a small child sit or pick up toys.

The same kind of faulty or inaccurate beliefs affect runners, too:

● Running is done with the legs. At first, this statement would seem so obvious as to border on the ridiculous. Of course we run with the legs! If we didn't have legs, we couldn't run. Consider, then, the view of Percy Cerutty, the late Australian Olympic coach, who said: 'You run on the legs, not with them.'

Runners who run with their legs tend to do more than is necessary in order to move. Rather than flowing, they do a lot of pushing and shoving, and their leg action lacks the fluidity and smoothness we see in great athletes or young children. They may push themselves upwards rather than rolling forwards, under the mistaken belief that running fast requires this kind of effort. They tend to focus only on contracting their legs rather than releasing into the front of the ankles and the backs of the knees, thereby forcing muscles to work against each other. They may pound, or run into the ground rather than over it, thereby contributing to the lower-leg problems that plague runners at all levels.

- The legs, and particularly the heels of the feet, should lead the movement. If a runner believes this (and it's not an uncommon idea, by the way), this tends to make the runner work against himself and fight against gravity rather than using it to his advantage. The runner will lean back and tighten in order not to fall, with his feet extending in front and pulling him along.

Five keys to running well

In contrast to these faulty and inaccurate beliefs, here are some of the key components in learning how to run well:

Good runners run tall

They don't hunch or lean. They run with the brakes off. There is an economy and integrity in their movement. They run smoothly. While it's true that the smoothest runner does not always get to the line first, good runners still represent the ideal to which we can aspire. As use improves, there should be a clear improvement in form: longer stride, longer spine, head not retracted, better use of the arms.

Less can equal more

Intelligent training means listening to your body, adapting your schedule to allow sufficient recovery and to maintain interest. It's not about following a programme blindly and irrationally, and disregarding pain. After all, the adaptations to the body caused by training occur when we rest, not when we are under the stress of exercise. By allowing adequate recuperation, our bodies recover, grow stronger and are less prone to breaking down. Coaches in all sports are now emphasizing the importance of quality rather than quantity as the key to improvement and greater all-round fitness.

Listen to the whispers so you won't have to hear the screams

Runners often train through and into injuries. Some must single-handedly keep pharmacists in business with their purchases of Vitamin I. A small niggle, if attended to, often disappears. This enables a runner to survive and even thrive on the stresses imposed by high-quality training. However, as the saying goes, 'Those who don't learn will be taught' – and the lesson can be very painful.

Runners who pound the ground often end up injured

Good runners run lightly; they don't try and excavate holes in the ground with each stride.

Have confidence in the process and enjoy it more

Alexander's belief that by paying attention to the means, the end would take care of itself, allowed me to take each day as it came when applied to the regimes of training and racing. I began to understand that I didn't need to put in extra workouts – and I started to see the tougher sessions, which could produce a lot of anxiety, as opportunities to learn. How should I react to the worry of striving for a particular target time, or cope with the pain this might cause? How should I enjoy the camaraderie of fellow runners, and take full satisfaction from completing something that seemed impossible half an hour earlier?

Why do we run badly?

In order to improve, it's essential to try hard. But this belief is often very effective at feeding the 'end-gaining' monster. As Percy Cerutty put it: 'The mind, drilled and grilled to wrong concepts, reacts against itself. The result is that as the athlete tries hard, the power exerted is transferred to his antagonistic muscles. The harder he tries, the more his brakes pull on.'

A simple definition of fanaticism is 'redoubling your efforts when you've lost sight of your goal'. Here are some signs that this may have happened:

- You work to the principle that 'more is more'. More mileage, more sessions, more effort, more vitamins, more shoes and, ultimately, more injuries.

- You ignore warning signs. You believe that 'no pain, no gain' is an ideal philosophy for training as well as for life. As for a cold, well, when did the snuffles ever keep you at home?

- You always run hard and compete whenever possible, especially in training. You try never to let anyone finish in front of you, even on 'easy' days.

- You train every day and never rest enough. You view walking, stopping to enjoy the view or to smell the flowers as signs of weakness.

- You become completely obsessed with having to run a certain distance or for a certain length of time each day and recording it in detail in your logbook. Not only that, you insist on telling anyone and everyone about it.

- As a 45-year-old male (replace age, sex, distance and goal to suit your own circumstances), your sense of well-being and personal esteem hinge on your breaking 47 mins for 10 km (6 miles).

Summary: running do's and don'ts

Do's

- Do allow the arms to engage the legs. The shoulders need to remain free so that the movement of the arms can connect with the legs through the back.

- Do allow the ankles to release, followed by a release towards the back of the knees. In order to allow the knees to bend freely – that is, without having to overcome any self-induced resistance – the ankles need to be free. Ask a friend to hold on to your ankle and try to bend your knee. You will need to work hard to overcome the resistance. When he lets go, the knees will bend much more easily. Any tension in the ankles will make a smooth stride much less likely.

- Do allow the knees, rather than the feet, to lead the movement forwards. Trying to increase stride length by reaching forward with the foot results in a braking action that will slow you down. It can also cause you to lean back or sit on your hips rather than run tall. Instead, let the knee lead the leg forwards, and stride length will come as a result of the foot extending behind you.

- Do focus on getting your feet off the ground. The less time they spend there, the better.

● Do remember that the external direction is forwards, and the internal direction is up. Many runners do not understand that although they may be moving forwards in space, their spine does not have to aim the same way. Ideally, as you are moving forwards (that is, horizontally) as a result of the action of your legs and feet, your spine should be lengthening upwards (that is, vertically), with the head leading the way. This upward tendency produces lightness in the body, which means that the legs do not have to work so hard to move you forward. When a runner's spine goes forwards instead of up, by pushing the chest or pelvis towards the target, it causes a downward shortening tendency in the back, as well as a feeling of heaviness. This is compensated for by the legs working much harder than they need to.

● Do let your eyes look out 30–50 m (98–164 ft) ahead. Not only will you see more of the countryside, cityscape or parkland, but running with a lengthened spine and a poised head will encourage balance and reduce both 'heavy' running and much of the strain on the neck and shoulders.

● Do allow the wrists to remain toned rather than floppy. Runners often mistakenly run with their wrists so loose that their hands flop around, in the belief that this helps them to be relaxed. They are, in fact, creating tension elsewhere, as the shoulders will often tighten to pick up the slack. Instead, runners should allow enough tone in their wrists to maintain a stable relationship between the hand and arm. Stiff thumbs are another indication that there is too much tension.

● Do allow the elbows to remain bent at 90 degrees. This is a very efficient way to organize the arms. While variations on this set-up are not a sin, remember that a short lever is more efficient as it requires less energy to move. Since we want the arms to contribute to the running action, we need to know how this can be done as effectively and smoothly as possible.

● Do allow the arms to move straight forward and back. Runners do a lot of interesting things with their arms. Some movements contribute more to propelling you forwards than others: the most effective is when the arms move forwards and back in a straight line. ('Arm' really means 'the upper arm'.) A sprinter's upper arm will be parallel to the ground both when it swings forwards and when it is pulled back. Runners moving less quickly should modify the range of motion to match their speed and terrain (less on the flat; more going uphill). Another point to note: the effort comes in pulling the arm back, not in pushing it forwards. Pulling the arm back helps the legs pull you forwards via the back.

- Do learn to run lightly and quietly. Pounding the ground is a sign that something's wrong. You may be tired, not feeling well or simply not paying attention. Running lightly has nothing to do with the amount you weigh: it has much more to do with attention (listening to yourself as you run) and intention (thinking 'up'). We continually need to ask ourselves which qualities support our capacity to make running a pleasure, and which do the opposite.

- Do run on the legs, not with the legs. This is Percy Cerutty's dictum. By overemphasizing the legs in running, an imbalance is created and overall coordination is compromised. The Italian concept, *appoggio*, normally used in the context of voice training, helps to explain what Cerutty means. *Appoggio* refers to our capacity to coordinate ourselves in such an efficient way that the function of one muscle is not violated by the exaggerated action of another. In other words, efficient running depends on our ability to coordinate the action of the legs with the seemingly 'inactive' upper body.

Don'ts

- Don't push the body up and let it land heavily on the legs with every stride. Pushing the body upwards takes a great deal of effort, which may be useful in a training context (to strengthen the legs, for example), but is an inefficient way to move a runner forwards. Some runners mistakenly believe that pushing themselves up with the legs helps them to run taller and faster. In fact, it tends to (a) stiffen the legs, (b) do little to increase overall height, which is a function of the length of the spine, and (c) waste valuable time and energy moving the body up against gravity. We're runners, not high jumpers.

- Don't push with the feet. Many runners think it necessary to push with the feet in order to run. This habit is unnecessary because there is plenty of friction between foot and ground (especially with today's high-tech shoes) to move the runner forwards without extra effort. Adding the push often interferes with coordination and puts strain on the foot, ankle and calf, which can lead to injury.

- Don't lock the arms on to the trunk or fix the shoulders. We often see runners who have allowed their arms to become heavy and unenergized, so they do not move as easily or freely as they should. The arms then function as weights, which serve to pull the runner down into a moving slouch. The problem does not necessarily originate with the arms, but can be traced back to a poor head-neck-back relationship. Thinking about freeing (not holding) the armpits can help release the arms and allow them to move more freely. This direction also helps to reduce the tension and pain in the shoulder blade and lower neck area that is suffered by some runners from time to time.

- Don't allow the feet to cross over the mid-line. Some runners like to let their feet cross over an imaginary line running between them, a habit that leads to the upper body swaying back and forth. This also throws the hips from side to side, as anyone who has seen or mimicked a model's catwalk stride will know. You then have to use extra effort and energy to adjust to all this lateral movement.

- Don't tuck or push the pelvis into the legs. Runners, especially those who arch their lower backs, are often advised to perform a 'pelvic tuck', where the buttocks are tightened and the pelvis is tucked under. The intention of this advice is to help reduce the excessive curve in the lower back. Unfortunately, this measure often causes unwanted side effects: for example, tucking the pelvis can produce a downward pull, which must be countered with muscular effort elsewhere, often in the form of pulling up the sternum. This tightens and narrows the lower back, fixes the ribs and makes it hard to breathe and to move the legs. In effect, a type of internal civil war is created, with one part of the body at odds with another: the pelvis trying to pull the back down and the sternum striving desperately to resist.

- Don't allow the head to roll, bob or wag. Once you are aware that the head weighs about 4.5 kg (10 lb), it's not hard to see that letting the head roll around is going to place a tremendous

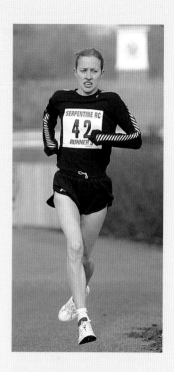

JULIA BLEASDALE ▲

A high-level runner and women's record holder for the Serpentine 5k race in London, Bleasdale shows how the demands of competition can exaggerate personal eccentricities – in her case, feet crossing over an imaginary line between them – otherwise known as 'misuse'. This demands extra energy and effort to adjust to the lateral movement.

load on the rest of the body, beginning with the spine. Runners who allow their head to wobble are often under the mistaken impression that this is a way to relax the neck. In reality, it puts more strain on the neck, which must now work much harder to cope with the constant shifts in the balance of the head.

- Don't allow the fists to clench, the wrists to flop or the thumbs to stiffen. Too much tension or not enough tone in the hands and wrists contributes to similar problems elsewhere.

- Don't clench the teeth or grimace. Runners can do some pretty awful things with their jaws, teeth and faces when they run, especially when under stress. Besides the possibility of frightening small children, facial grimaces do little to help you get from A to B. In fact, they can be an indication that your energy is being misdirected rather than going to where it will do most good.

- Don't bounce up and down or roll from side to side. Research has shown that elite runners have less vertical change in their centre of mass compared to average runners, and that reducing one's quantity of vertical movement tends to improve running economy.

- Don't push the chest towards the target. When you do this, the head tends to be thrown backwards – away from the target! Pushing or lifting the chest also tightens and hollows the back, which makes it harder to breathe naturally and leads to the following suggestion: belly breathing. Try to remember our first principle: the head leads and the body follows.

- Don't belly breathe. Some coaches advocate belly breathing as the correct way to breathe when running. While the technique of slow breathing from the diaphragm may be useful in meditation and as a way to lessen the symptoms of anxiety and panic, it's actually of little use to runners. However, it is safe to say that if you try to run tall by lifting your chest, tucking your pelvis and thereby fixing your ribs, you may not have any option but to belly breathe! For proof, hold your lower ribs firmly with your hands and try to take a deep breath. You'll find that it's not easy. Now try slumping and taking a deep breath. The same thing will happen. In these circumstances, the runner's only option for gaining a full breath is to over-expand the abdomen.

AFTERWORD
Centred running

Unlike the dancer, the runner has no intention to be self-expressive.
Nonetheless, the running self is always self-expressive. A contemporary
lifestyle that is pulled by the nose into the future and pushed in the back
by the past expresses itself in a running style that thrusts out the
advancing leg, taking a 'footful' of ground and pushing it from behind.
Looked at from the point of balance, it is clear that balance is impossible
with a leg stuck out in front or behind. The crucial point in the running
cycle happens when the supporting leg is directly beneath the body's
centre. Here the body regains balance.

A runner who commits to the process of centring will not be pulled by
the future or pushed by the past. Only in the present moment can the
runner's gaze move beyond the 'end-gaining' one of win/lose. Self-
discovery unfolds from the centre. The centred runner moves wholly into
the present moment, at one with himself or herself, each running step
merging into a oneness with the ground. The centred runner is aware of
the questions 'Where am I going?' and 'Where have I been?', but
constantly returns to the key question: 'Where am I now?'

With eyes lifted to the wider horizon of self-discovery, the centred
runner naturally attends to the core issues of balance, alignment,
suspension and graceful release. *John Woodward*

BIBLIOGRAPHY

Further information

Since I first came into contact with Alexander Technique in 1979, the number of books on the subject has grown enormously. At that time, the only readily available books were Dr Wilfred Barlow's *The Alexander Principle* and Edward Maisel's *The Resurrection of the Body*. I can remember scouring second-hand bookshops and market stalls in and around London in the vain hope of finding a copy of one of Alexander's original four volumes. The situation today is very different: all of Alexander's works have been reprinted. In addition, the website www.alexandertech.com offers a selection of articles.

Recommended DVD on running

Evolution Running DVD (Velo Press)
An excellent video on improving your running.

Recommended books on the Alexander Technique

Pedro de Alcantara: *The Alexander Technique: A Skill For Life* (Crowood Press, 1999) This is an excellent introductory text.

F. Matthias Alexander: *The Use of the Self* (Integral Press, 1955)

Michael Gelb: *Body Learning* (Aurum Press, 1994)

Frank Pierce Jones: *Body Awareness in Action* (Schoken Books, 1979)

Patrick Macdonald: *The Alexander Technique As I See It* (Rahula Books, 1989)

Edward Maisel (Ed): *The Resurrection of the Body* (Shambhala Books, 1986)

Steven Shaw and Armand D'Angour: *The Art of Swimming* (Ashgrove Press, 1996)

Jerry Sontag (Ed): *Curiosity Recaptured* (Mornum Time Press, 1996)

Recommended books on running

Percy Wells Cerutty: Athletics: *How to Become a Champion* (Sportsmans Book Club, 1961) Hard to find but worth looking for.

Sebastian and Peter Coe: *Running For Fitness* (Sphere Books, 1983)

Bob Cooley: *The Genius of Flexibility* (Fireside, 2005) Stretching with a difference!

Jack Daniels: *Daniels' Running Formula* (Human Kinetics, 1998)

John Douillard: *Body, Mind and Sport* (Crown Trade Paperbacks, 1994)

Danny Dreyer: *Chi Running* (Simon & Schuster, 2004) A well-written book. Similar to the Pose Method, but with an emphasis on eastern philosophy. Lots of good tips for beginners.

Jeff Galloway: *Galloway's Book On Running* (Shelter Publications, 1984)

Bernd Heinrich: *Why We Run* (Harper Collins, 2002) A lyrical and scientific exploration of running interwoven with the author's quest to set the 100k world record. What a book; what a runner!

Frank Horwill: *Obsession For Running* (Colin Davis, 1991) Written by a rare and unique personality and coach.

John Jerome: *Staying With It* (Breakaway Books, 1968) A gem for ageing warrior-athletes.

John Jerome: *The Sweet Spot in Time* (Summit Books, 1980) A straightforward yet beautifully written book on the physiology of training.

WR Loader: *Testament of a Runner* (Kingswood Press, 1960) Classic account of competing in the 1950s.

Dr Jerry Lynch: *The Total Athlete* (Prentice-Hall, 1987)

Dr Jerry Lynch and Warren Scott: *Running Within* (Human Kinetics, 1999) A guide to mastering the body-mind-spirit connection for ultimate training and racing.

Brent McFarlane: *The Science of Hurdling* (Canadian Track and Field Association, 1988)

Kenny Moore: *Best Efforts* (Cedarwinds Publishing, 1982)

Tim Noakes: *The Lore of Running* (Oxford University Press, 2003)

Roy Palmer: *The Performance Paradox* (Delaney & Smith, 2001) A challenge to conventional methods of sports training and exercise by an Alexander Technique teacher and athlete.

John L Parker Jr: *Once A Runner* (Cedarwinds Publishing, 1978) The greatest book ever written on running!

John L Parker Jr: *Runners and Other Dreamers* (Cedarwinds Publishing, 1989)

Dr Nicholas Romanov: *Pose Method of Running* (Pose Tech Press, 2002) Controversial, thought-provoking, revolutionary and well-written. Definitely worth a read.

Dr Nicholas Romanov: *Strength Conditioning, Hip and Hamstring Exercises* (Pose Tech Press, 2002) If you're looking for drills and want to try something different, this book is filled with challenging and rewarding exercises for runners at all levels.

Michael Sandrock: *Running With the Legends* (Human Kinetics, 1996)

George Sheehan: *Running To Win* (Rodale Press, 1992)

Mel C Siff: *Facts and Fallacies of Fitness* (Self-published, 1998)

Liz Sloan and Ann Kramer: *Running: the Women's Handbook* (Pandora Press, 1985)

Useful contacts

The Society of Teachers of the Alexander Technique, 20 London House, 266 Fulham Road, London SW10 9EL (020 7351 0828 www.stat.org.uk).

The Art of Running: for information about workshops in the UK, Canada, USA and elsewhere, visit www.theartofrunning.com.

The Art of Swimming: for information about Steven Shaw's workshops in the UK and overseas, visit www.artofswimming.com.

Terry Fox: to find out about the inspirational figure to whom this book is dedicated and take part in one of the runs, in more than 50 countries, that bear his name to raise money for cancer research, visit www.terryfoxrun.org.

INDEX

Picture credits

page 2 Richard Dunkley
pages 4-5, 7, 55, 57, 59, 69, 70, 75, 76, 79, 87, 89,
91, 95, 96, 97, 139 Guy Hearn
pages 10 REUTERS/Mike Blake, 26 REUTERS/Brian
Snyder, 112 REUTERS/Carlos Barria, 122
REUTERS/Pascal Lauener, 125 REUTERS/Jerry
Lampen
pages 25 Jean Guichard/Sygma/CORBIS, 37 Norbert
Schaefer/CORBIS, 51 Dan Helms/NewSport/Corbis,
93, 99 Bettmann/CORBIS, 128 Thierry Orban/Corbis
page 35 Tom Blau/Camera Press, London
pages 40, 117, 119, 131 Empics
page 73 Reuters/Corbis

pages 77, 102 Gary Hershorn/Reuters/Corbis
page 82 Yves Herman
page 114 Sandra Boynton, excerpted from 'One, Two,
Three!', used by permission of Workman Publishing Co
Inc
pages 132-133 Claus Anderson
page 152 David Knight